# 50 BEST YOGA POSITIONS

A step-by-step guide to the best exercises for mind, body, and soul

First published by Parragon in 2011

Parragon
Chartist House
15-17 Trim Street
Bath BA1 1HA, UK
www.parragon.com

Designed by Stonecastle Graphics Limited
Compiled by Gillian Haslam
© Getty Images: pages 7, 9, 12, 13, 17ar, 19, 69, 95, 103 and 145.
© Shutterstock.com: Yuri Arcurs 85; Phil Date 27, 49; Yellowj 11.
Cover Images: *Top left, middle smaller image:* Forward Bend Yoga
Position © John Freeman/Getty Images. *Top left, third smaller
image:* Woman Stretching © Jack Wild/Getty Images. *Top right:*
Woman Meditating © Image Source/Getty Images. *Bottom left,
top image:* Fish Yoga Pose © John Freeman/Getty Images.
*All other cover images:* © iStock

ISBN: 978-1-4454-5389-7

Printed in China

Note:
As a precautionary measure, the publishers advise that anyone
intending to follow the exercise programs outlined in this book
should first consult a qualified practitioner or therapist.

# 50 BEST YOGA POSITIONS

A step-by-step guide to the best exercises for mind, body, and soul

## PaRragon

Bath · New York · Singapore · Hong Kong · Cologne · Delhi
Melbourne · Amsterdam · Johannesburg · Auckland · Shenzhen

# CONTENTS

*Left:* Matsyasana
(see *page 78*).

# INTRODUCTION

After their first yoga class, people often report that they've slept better and feel taller. Yoga has helped people lose weight, overcome fears, conquer habits like smoking and develop better concentration, all of which help their performance in daily tasks. Others feel improved self-awareness, a deeper sense of wellbeing, developed compassion, enhanced relationships, greater self-acceptance, and a sensation of being at peace.

As we nudge our physical boundaries with yoga postures, we become fully focused on body, breath, and mind. We become absorbed in being in the present moment. It's a break from our usual mind status; it refreshes us. Yoga practice helps us move from distress to de-stress, from dis-ease to ease, from passion to compassion.

Contrary to what many believe, yoga is not a set of exercises or a meditation technique. It is actually a state of mind. The state of yoga is when the mind is still. The turnings of thoughts have ceased and there are no distractions. Over the last 2,000 years, other practices were developed that helped the body and mind become receptive to the experience of stillness. Of these practices, asana (physical postures) is the practice most commonly equated with yoga in the West. Stillness fosters awareness. Hatha yoga includes physical exercises that seek to relax and still the body, breath work to focus the mind, relaxation to quieten the body and mind, chanting to arouse and then calm the emotions, and meditation to center the spirit.

The word yoga originates from the Sanskrit word *yuj*. Yuj may be translated as "to center one's thoughts" or "to meditate deeply," both of which involve the slowing of the movements of the mind. From yuj also comes to "unite" and "connect," which imply a reintegration, a bringing back into balance. It is often said that yoga means union, as it harmonizes body, breath, mind and spirit. But, paradoxically, yoga also seeks to disunite. The spirit, considered pure and eternal, separates from the physical body, and its purity is regained. Lastly, from the root yuj comes "to yoke."Yoking, or harnessing one's energies, connotes effort, and Hatha Yoga certainly requires this. The codes of moral conduct, physical exercises, breathing practices, concentration, and meditation all require effort, and all contribute to the goal of self-realization. Keeping a healthy discipline makes life feel better. Sometimes you begin your practice feeling unfocused, lethargic, anxious, or tight in your body. Yet after absorbing yourself in your practice, you feel warm, loose, relaxed, calm, and perhaps more connected to a force greater than you.

Being off balance doesn't feel good—it's difficult to relate to others in a relaxed, authentic way. Fear fades and tranquillity arrives when you relax back into a sense of wholeness. It's when you re-remember who you are.

When you practice yoga, you might spend 30 minutes on the mat twice a week, or you might expand it into your way of life. When you are right there in the moment, there is nothing to work toward, and, as you mentally sink into that moment, worries fall away. Yoga lets us practice being in the present. The reality is that the present moment is all we really possess.

*Right:* Yoga harmonizes body, breath, mind, and spirit.

# THE ASANAS

Watching my cats wake up is a lesson in itself. They reach forward and stretch back just like the yoga pose of Downward-Facing Dog. Then they round their backs while arching up (which we call Cat Pose) and yawn. Slow stretching is glorious. It feels good and the body likes it. Our body wants to move and was designed for it. It feels better to be loose and free than to be all bound up, tense and contracted.

A yoga "asana" is a posture where you are externally still, yet internally alive. To take part in asana practice is to use your body as the doorway through which to experience and remember the truth about who you are. By holding an asana we can integrate the body, breath, and mind.

One of the most common mental blocks for a beginner is the belief that they are not flexible enough for yoga. Advanced practitioners make the action look effortless. Many of the photos in this book are of teachers who have many years of asana practice. Mostly, the fullest forms of the asanas are shown. This is meant to inspire you, not discourage you!

As long as your alignment is not harming your body, it is not important whether your pose looks graceful. What matters is that you find the teaching point for that pose. It may be that, due to your body's individuality, you need to change the posture to fit you, rather than overriding the body's needs by forcing it to conform to an "ideal" shape. More than poise in the posture, it is the breath that should be graceful.

According to the Yoga-Sutra, the first codification of yoga, which dates back about 2,000 years, an asana must have the qualities of alertness and relaxation. It is perfected when no effort is necessary, hence relaxation is possible. Even if you feel like you have the flexibility of a block of wood, keep in mind the concept of "abhyasa" or "repeated effort." With repeated effort you cease to have to try.

Asanas help balance the body. They distribute strength and flexibility evenly between left and right, top and bottom, front and back. They develop strength in weaker areas of the body, and softness in tighter spots. Through freeing up the outer body, asanas build and control the "prana"—the vital force—in the inner body. On an energetic level, polarity therapists believe the joints in the body can be weaker areas, and yoga postures mobilize and vitalize the joints.

Asanas focus the mind and are a way of coming back to the self. Like your body finding its center of gravity in a given position, finding just where your center is in your life is helpful. Asanas teach you that moving away from your center only creates internal conflict. Becoming stiller, and therefore more aware, with yoga practice helps you notice when you are moving away from your center so you have the chance to bring yourself back.

***Above:*** *The ancient texts tell us that the state of yoga can be reached through dedication and practice.*

# THE BREATH

Your breath will bring your yoga alive. When you are consciously breathing, your practice can never be mechanical. Good breathing is reassuring, soothing, and healing. It will bring intuition to your postures. Remember that even in the seemingly stationary poses when your body might be still on the outside, it is never stagnant. While there is breath awareness, there will be a feeling of cleansing, lightness, new energy, and mental clarity. If you forget your "breath" then come back to an exercise where the breath and movement are clearly linked so that you feel the flow. Holding the breath dulls the flow of feeling. If your breath freezes, ease the intensity of your posture, let the rhythm into the belly and chest once more, and catch the wave of the breath when it comes.

The breath is a mirror for your mind. Breath and mind are intrinsically connected. Any alteration in one will affect the other. The mind can multiply in ways that the breath cannot. As the breath is the slower moving of the two, choosing to focus on it during asana practice will help to calm the churnings of thought. Awareness of the breath will draw your mind to the present moment. Evenness in your breath will be reflected in your mind. The breath is your monitor of how you are doing in the pose. When the breath flows steadily, your asana becomes closer to being perfected.

Your natural breath can't be created by willpower alone. You can breathe freely only through releasing and undoing. The natural breath unshrinks and unkinks us and teaches us that sometimes the most subtle methods are the most profound. Come back to the breath often throughout the day and check how you are breathing.

Breathe in and out through the nose so that the air is filtered and warmed. To bring constancy to your breath, practice yoga asanas with a steady breath. In general, inhale on opening or unfolding the body, when performing rising-up or lengthening movements, when twisting the upper back, and when bending backward. Exhale when releasing, closing the body, moving downward, twisting the lower back, lowering the arms or legs, and when bending forward or sideways. These are general rules but do experiment to intuit what feels right for your body.

Try a practice moving only on the exhalation, for example. The slower you move, the more easily awareness will come. In flowing postures, experiment with taking three or five breaths to complete a single movement. Remind yourself that it's irrelevant whether you can touch your toes or not. If you can breathe, you can practice yoga.

# STAYING PRESENT

When you stay mentally present in a pose, awareness deepens. There are two types of asanas: conscious and unconscious. In a conscious position, the quality of the asana moves from that of body conditioner to become a psycho-spiritual exercise. When you are absorbed in the subtle sensations of the body, your mind is not permitted to dance away. Your mind will naturally run to the part of your body where the feelings are intense, but try to spread your awareness simultaneously and evenly over your body. From observing your hamstring in a forward bend, radiate your awareness to the whole leg, then keep radiating it out until it touches the entire body.

If you spend one minute in a posture, observe, sense, visualize, and refine. Seek that still point, the epicenter of consciousness. Over the duration of your practice, these "one minutes" join together to create a unit of time during which you have been perfectly present. These blocks of time are healing and refreshing.

# DOING AND UNDOING

Fully engaging a muscle will bring the mind right to that area. All-over awareness is excellent practice for concentration and being in the now. With the muscles engaged, the mind is engaged and this is why yoga asanas have transformative power.

According to the Yoga-Sutra, an asana needs to be steady and comfortable. The stretching of yoga aims to expand, not strain. Strain blocks your ability to listen to what the body has to tell you. Go to the deepest you can, then hold it a little bit more. Non-harming is one of the precepts of yoga philosophy, and this certainly includes your treatment of your body. Overworking

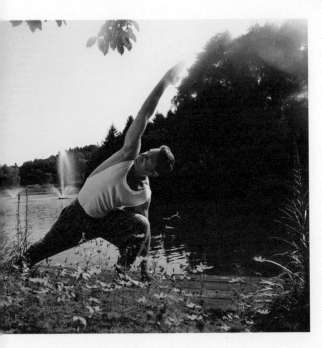

slow rhythmic movement may help. Flow in and out of the pose several times, before finally holding the pose. As you release the air from your lungs, release the tension in the body. Don't force, simply yield with each exhalation to extend further. Let tension move out of your body and into the atmosphere.

## ANCHORING AND RADIATING

With yoga, as in life, we need a base from which to move. When we are stable and grounded, directional movement can be focused. While one part of your body is well grounded, another part can rise up. When you anchor yourself securely, it makes the exercise more of a challenge. Often, less flexible people have a better yoga practice than those who are very flexible. Stiffer-bodied people know intuitively about anchoring and working from their base. People who are naturally flexible have to learn how to anchor themselves. Having a point from which to extend yourself is physiologically a bit like using weights in a gym. As you engage your muscles, there is a point from which to work.

Consider where your anchor is in each pose. The floor acts as your base when standing. As you take your arms overhead, extend and radiate upward from floor to fingertips. When you sit to bend forward, ground down through the sitting bones. When you lie prone to backbend, press down through the pubic bone and radiate out from the lower abdomen. When you sit to twist right, anchor the left buttock well down. In Shoulderstand, let the shoulders and elbows be heavy so the rest of the body can float lightly upward. When you hold your arms horizontal and stretch them apart, radiate your energy along the arms and reach outward, so it feels like it is not just your muscular power holding them in place, but your mental energy stretching them away.

Our center of gravity lies 2 in (5 cm) below the navel. Learn to move from this center. This core acts as an anchor from which to extend. Then the movement from the center to the extremities feels integrated, and ripples of energy flow from our center to the rest of the body. Link them with the breath, the extension outward and the gentle rebounding flow back. Practice extending yourself without losing yourself.

your body is neglecting to take care, a form of misuse. Coax and persuade but don't force.

Some days it feels hard to pull yourself up out of your armchair. Other days you effortlessly spring up. When you engage the mind in the posture, you give strength to the posture. With strength comes a lovely feeling of lightness, too. It's like changing from a heavy, old car to a new one with power steering. When you have energy, strength, and lightness, it's much more pleasurable to move your body around.

Upon first meeting a posture, it might feel that it requires 100 percent effort to hold it. It can be hard to imagine being able to find any release in the pose at all. As you practice and become more comfortable with the pose, the effort required slowly reduces. With time and dedication, the proportion of doing to undoing will slide. The asana will feel more comfortable and more rewarding. Freedom comes into the pose.

We are accustomed to the concept of using effort to get somewhere. Letting go in order to achieve something might seem strange. Counter the effort of doing with plenty of undoing. Do more by doing less. If you are standing, enjoy the relief in surrendering your weight down through the soles of the feet. If you are sitting, sink down through the sitting bones. If you are balancing on your hands, soften the skin on the palms and release downward. This downward energy rebounds upward to be used in your posture. If the release won't come in a posture,

*Above left and opposite:* Yoga positions bring strength to weak areas of the body.

# BANDHAS

A "bandha" involves the contraction of certain muscles to unlock the pranic vital energies so it can be directed upward. Bandhas may be used in conjunction with pranayama or asana practice to encourage the flow of the vital force and preserve it.

The bandhas are very useful during asana practice. They work with the organs, and the nervous and endocrine systems. They can improve disorders of the reproductive and urinary systems, sexual dysfunction and back problems, and are helpful in the alleviation of problems experienced after childbirth.

The mulabandha is located at the perineum—the area between the anus and the genitals, and about 1 in (2.5 cm) in toward the core of the body. For women, it is also linked to the cervix. Uddhyanabandha is located in the core of the body just below the navel.

To practice with mulabandha and uddhyanabandha, sit erect. On your next inhalation, draw in the lower abdomen—the part just above the pubic bone and below the navel. As you do this, the perineum will lift slightly and a gentle mulabandha holding will be activated. Move between drawing in on the inhalation and letting go on the exhalation, so you get a sense of the lifting sensation in the pelvis.

When you are not used to isolating the mulabandha area, the surrounding muscles seem to want to tense up in sympathy. You might find your buttocks, thighs, and anus tightening, or that you are unconsciously holding your breath. In time, you will be able to more actively draw up the perineum without tensing other muscles.

The bandhas respond to different parts of the breath—while drawing in the lower abdomen is easiest on the inhalation, you might notice that actively drawing up the perineum feels easiest on an exhalation. Practice this while sitting, then incorporate it into forward bends and standing poses. Eventually, bring it into the other poses, too.

*Above: During your practice you will experience strong sensations.*

# DISCOMFORT AND PAIN

During your practice you will feel intense sensations. The sensations you get from a strong stretch are not necessarily bad. You might feel discomfort, which is a "good hurt," or pain, a "negative hurt." Discomfort is resistance of the body or mind. When exploring new territory, mental and physical unease will inevitably arise.

Pain is more acute than discomfort. Discomfort, when caused by working strongly, is a positive feeling. With pain, there will be nothing pleasant about the soreness. Pain in a pose means you have overshot your limit by moving too quickly, or that you are improperly aligned. Pain is counterproductive as the body will instinctively tense and move away from it. Pain in the muscles or joints could lead to injury, so never ignore it. Come out of the pose and examine your alignment or check with a teacher.

A high strain will force your attention away, while, if you are underworking your body, the mind will become lethargic. Optimum strain, working just at your edge, will engage your mind. When your body experiences a healthy amount of tension, you can move internally and tune into the quietness. Remember that yoga seeks to remove pain and suffering, not increase it.

# YOUR EDGE

Your edge is the point at which the strong challenge comes into the pose and where you feel you have reached a new frontier. During practice, aim to push back your edge in a slow, respectful way. Listen to your body's feedback, not only immediately after practice but over the following days. Each pose has many edges; each one is an opportunity to grow. As you approach your first edge, hold the position with a steady breath. Stay focused on that place in your body. Exhalation will help soften and prepare the body to move beyond it. Wait for your body to let you in. Should that inner cue come, proceed respectfully, with full attention. Then you have found a new edge. Likewise, it is good to be adventurous but this does not mean you should be aggressive.

the process. Yoga asanas are a controlled means of exposing yourself to a difficult situation. They are meant to challenge you. They offer practice at mastering your reaction under stressful conditions. If you experience mental unease, absorb yourself in the breath. Should you find you are in a place that feels wrong, change it. If either your body or mind is telling you "no," don't push past it. Instead, as you do whenever circumstances change in your life, adjust. Be mentally flexible, too. Sensitively encourage yourself using your breath, but never force it.

## YOUR INTENTION

Consider what you want to achieve with yoga. You might want to increase strength or flexibility, heal an ailment, find better body awareness, cope with stress, find inner peace, develop compassion, or explore your spirituality. Write down what it is you want so that you will be clear and can form your practice around your goal. Also write how much time you can realistically expect to practice.

Yoga is not religious. Though yoga has been embraced by Hinduism, as they are both from Indian soil, there is nothing in the yoga texts that speak of Hinduism. The writings do, however, recognize a divine principle, a universal energy. If you have a religious tradition that you find helpful, keep your personal god in mind. If not, consider your higher goals, or ideals that inspire you. Keeping an energy greater than ourselves in mind fosters our ability to attune to our higher self.

At the start of your practice you might like to light a candle or an incense stick, offer a chant or prayer, or repeat an affirmation. You might look at a picture of your personal god, or a photo of someone inspirational with qualities you admire. Take time at the beginning to sit or lie quietly and access the stillness within. Be clear of your intent, but begin each practice with an open mind. Yoga, stilling the fluctuations of the mind, is an end point, but your practice is part of your journey, and a reward in itself.

Be clear that this is time for you alone. Close the door and turn off the phone. Let others know not to distract you. When a posture feels cumbersome and heavy, it will be less enjoyable. Bring mental lightness to your practice, too—enthusiasm always lightens the load. Practice with renewed effort when you feel lazy. If you feel you are a Type A overachiever, learn to ease off when your body requires it. Work honestly, with integrity, curiosity, and enthusiasm. Be joyful in your practice.

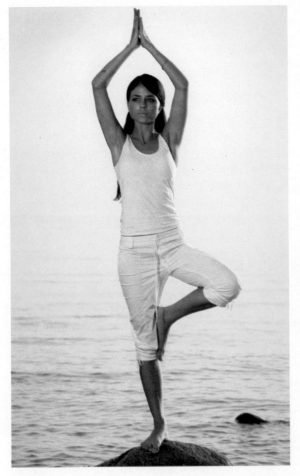

*Above: Begin each practice with an open mind and be clear that this is time for you alone.*

Your body is constantly responding to other circumstances. Just where your edge is varies from breath to breath, practice to practice, day to day. Rediscover your limit in every pose. Never take it for granted that you can stretch as far as you did yesterday. Never assume that you can't because you couldn't before.

It's irrelevant where your edge is in an asana. It is unimportant how far you stretch before you find it. Whether you reach your fingertips to your knees as you fold forward or whether you easily grasp your feet, let go of preconceptions of "good" or "proper" yoga. Seek instead just to find the point where you can learn about yourself.

Your psychological edge might be different to your physical edge. Respect both. Yoga should help you deal with life, not hinder

# PHILOSOPHY

Hatha yoga consists of eight limbs of practices. They are not steps to be worked on one by one, but branches that can be explored, many at a time.

## 1 THE YAMAS

The "yamas" guide us in how we relate to others, our actions, thoughts and speech. There are five listed in the Yoga-Sutra:

### Ahimsa: Consideration for All Living Things

Often translated as non-violence, ahimsa encompasses compassion for all beings. As well as obvious things like not killing insects or being abusive, this includes subtle things, such as avoiding gossip and mastering negative thoughts. Protect the environment by respecting nature and recycling. Develop kindness, patience, and tolerance for others and for yourself. Incorporate ahimsa in the way you eat and choose nourishing foods.

### Satya: Right Communication

"Satya" deals with truthfulness and honesty in behavior and thought. It means restraining from deceptions or making a promise you cannot keep. If tempted to tell a "white" lie, be honest about your motivation. Is it to protect another or due to your inability to face an awkward situation? Lack of truth in any relationship doesn't build a stable foundation. Our task is to approach life with integrity and sincerity.

### Asteya: Non-Covetousness

Despite its translation as non-stealing, "asteya" encompasses resisting the desire for things that don't belong to us, to avoid living in a state of unfulfilled wanting. Enjoy the simpler gifts of life. Asteya includes not taking that which is not freely given, such as not stealing another person's time by being late or bullying someone into providing you with something you want. It means not "taking" the partner of another in an extramarital affair. Asteya encompasses giving credit where it is due.

### Brahmacharya: Moderation in Our Actions

This has many interpretations, one of which is celibacy. Many spiritual traditions preach celibacy not because they consider sex is bad, but so that energies can be used to uplift "the Self." Celibacy as a tool for discovering oneself can be a joyous, self-nurturing experience. An interpretation of "brahmacharya" might be being moderate in thoughts and actions. Channeling your sexuality with thought helps you to respect its power and use it with love.

### Aparigraha: Non-Greediness

Consider your true needs—the less you need, the greater chance you have of being happy. Practice simplicity by paring down possessions to the essentials. Downsize the spiral of want and enjoy what you already have. Consider how easily you give to others. Appreciate that which is around you—good food, your health, uplifting conversation, a good friend.

## 2 THE NIYAMAS

The second limb, "niyamas," deals with our attitudes toward ourselves. The Yoga-Sutra lists five:

### Saucha: Purity

"Saucha" is cleanliness of your physical body and surroundings. As mind and body influence each other, a healthy diet contributes to purity of the mind. Purity in your home means not cluttering it with possessions. Cleanliness of living encompasses what you say, read and watch on TV, and who you associate with. Yoga cleanses the body with postures and breathing techniques. Clearing the mind through observance of the yamas and niyamas, and cleansing the spirit with meditation, allows for clarity of thinking.

### Santosha: Contentment

Cultivate being satisfied with what you have, such as the knowledge that your basic needs are met, wonderful memories, your friendships and your health. Appreciating these things helps to bring the happiness we seek. "Santosha" cultivates an uncomplaining approach toward what you don't have, rather than accepting what you have because you are too lazy to change. Embrace inner growth.

### Tapas: Burning Enthusiasm

"Tap" means "to burn" or "to cook." Under this precept, you cook the raw ingredients of which you are composed to produce a beautiful dish. Tapas involves the self-control to live with good habits in all things including work, food, drink, spirituality, thoughts, and wishes. Bring enthusiasm to all parts of your life and stay focused on your spiritual path.

### Swadhyaya: Self-Study

Self-discovery demands a turning of the attention inward. Observe your responses under all circumstances. Whether you are relaxed or stressed, happy or sad, practice mindful self-reflection. Many people find keeping a journal helpful as a way of evaluating progress. Some choose therapy on their path to self-discovery; others attend spiritual classes. Read uplifting literature and other yoga books. As well as drawing your attention inward, extend your mind with philosophy and other studies that help you understand the world.

### Ishvarapranidhana: Celebration of the Spiritual

Here we accept the existence of a higher intelligence. By honoring our relation to this all-knowing principle we surrender our small ego before a higher will, helping to fulfill our destiny. Remember this omnipresent force always lies within. If you don't have a personal god, you may wish to celebrate an ideal.

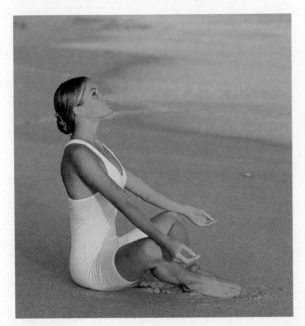

## 3 ASANA  Postures

"Asana," the third limb of yoga, is using physical postures as a method of self-study and exploration. Asana prepares the body and mind for meditation.

## 4 PRANAYAMA  Control of the Prana

While breath comes automatically and unconsciously, "pranayama"is the conscious, deliberate regulation of the breath and prana, the vital force.

## 5 PRATYAHARA  Withdrawal of the Senses

An example of this is when your hearing switches off from a dripping tap because you are engrossed in a book. While the senses are outward looking, self-discovery involves turning the attention inward, subduing the senses. Listen to less radio and watch less TV; practice deep relaxation and meditation.

## 6 DHARANA  Concentration

To maintain a mind undisturbed in its focus requires a certain mastery. Start small. Divide your dharana practice into small blocks of time—perhaps 30 seconds in an asana when you direct your mind to your body. During pranayama, direct it exclusively to the breath. By practicing you will become more accomplished.

## 7 DHYANA  Meditation

"Dhyana" is a one-pointed mental focus around a single subject.

## 8 SAMADHI  Bliss State

The highest level of experience and the goal of yoga—a bliss state where there is a sense of oneness. You reconnect with your essential purity, yet personal identity is not lost. The mind is mastered and thoughts are stilled in this trancelike state.

**Left:** *Through yoga, the body attains attractiveness to others, beauty, firmness, and unusual physical strength.*

# THE PRACTICE

# STARTING THE JOURNEY

The following guidelines will help you get more out of your practice. Creating a special yoga practice area will reaffirm your commitment. You don't need much space, but make sure the area is warm, clean, and uncluttered.

Choose non-restrictive clothes that you feel good in. Dress in layers to remain comfortable throughout your practice. Bare feet are best—wear socks only when your feet are cold. Intense practice in direct sunlight tends to be fatiguing, but relaxing in its warmth at the end is lovely. Practicing outside lets you commune with nature, but it can be more distracting than staying inside. It's a great idea to invest in a yoga mat. Apart from providing cushioning and a non-slip surface, it will make your mental commitment to your practice stronger. You will feel you can create a yoga space anywhere, simply by rolling out your mat.

Yoga works with prana, the vital force. Asana and pranayama practice bring this energy to the cells so they receive nourishment, and can perform their functions and heal. When you eat, your energies are made available to the digestive system in preference to the other systems. So after a meal, leave a space before you practice. Wait one hour after having a piece of fruit or a juice. Wait three or four hours after a large meal. Hydrate yourself beforehand so you don't disturb yourself during the practice.

Be realistic when you decide how much time you would like to, and are able to, dedicate to your practice. It is helpful to make a mental commitment. Do your best to stick to it, but don't think unkindly about yourself if you take a break. There has never been a yoga mat that has laid a guilt trip on someone who didn't use it for a while! Just work from where you are today. When you are short of time, practicing fewer poses with complete attention is preferable to rushing through many poses. From time to time, look through the book to check on the exercises you might have been avoiding. Try to embrace them into your practice.

You don't need three-hour-long sessions of complicated asanas to practice "real" yoga. Sometimes one instant or a single breath is all you need to reconnect with yourself. Yoga practice is more than what you do on the mat. It is about how you live your life once you step off it, and that's 24 hours a day.

There are thousands of variations on hundreds of yoga poses, but don't let this intimidate you. Even if you feel like a human ironing board, you can benefit enormously from about 20 poses practiced regularly. It's like tending a garden. Left uncared for, the soil starts to dry up and the plants start to wither. Once the garden has got to a certain state, it's too late to rush in with the big hoses. Large amounts of water might be more than it can readily accept, and instead it needs the kindness of water given little and often. If you have neglected your internal garden for a while, you'll need to practice in small, regular doses for it to grow and thrive.

Rather than focus on "perfecting" a posture as your measure of success in yoga, enjoy discovering your body and mind. Yoga is like life. It's a journey. Every yoga practice you have will be different, as you respond to internal and external conditions. Your thoughts change in a fraction of a second. The breath alters from second to second. How far you can stretch or hold a pose changes from minute to minute.

Empty your mind so that you can fully absorb the lessons of your practice. You never can predict just what they will be. If you are more adept, don't assume because you have practiced a posture a hundred times that you know everything about it. Keep the mind receptive and open to learning. Don't be impatient in your practice. Practice peacefully. Keep your mind sensitive. Overstraining the body will lessen your mental sensitivity. Some days you just might not feel like getting on your mat or doing breath work. Instead, your yoga practice might include reading something spiritually uplifting.

Take things easy during menstruation. It's a special time when it is nice to allow your energies to go inside. Avoid strong backbends and strong twists. Inverted postures make the flow have to work against gravity, so avoid them. Women have a natural body clock that reminds them to practice slow, restful yoga regularly, but in my classes, men are allowed to "menstruate," too!

While yoga has helped the pregnancies and labors of countless women, it is not safe to begin during the first three months of pregnancy. Many poses need to be modified so it's best to attend specialized classes during the second and third trimesters.

If you are suffering from a health condition or have an injury, seek guidance from an experienced yoga teacher or yoga therapist. Don't practice asanas or pranayama if you have a fever.

Attend some yoga classes. Yoga is so personal that each teacher will have something different to offer you. Teachers can give valuable feedback on your alignment and ideas for practice. Try teachers from several different traditions of yoga to find what suits you. Most yoga schools offer beginners' courses.

**Above:** Practicing outside lets you commune with nature but may be more distracting than staying inside.

**Right and opposite:** Don't be impatient. Practice peacefully and keep your mind sensitive.

# YOGA RELAXATION

Center yourself with a short relaxation before starting your asana practice, and always use it at the end of your practice. The final relaxation allows your body to integrate and consolidate the effects of the poses.

Imagine driving your car along the highway at high speed, for weeks on end. What would happen if you stopped only briefly to check the oil and water and refill the fuel? How long would your car last if subjected to days, weeks, and years of this? Now consider how you are driving your body. Like your car, your body will run better if given high-quality fuel and regular tune-ups. It will perform better for you when allowed to cool down with regular rest breaks.

Yoga asanas stir up the subtle energies (prana) of the body and the relaxation is the time that allows the prana to be directed to healing and re-energizing the system. You might feel like nothing is happening and be tempted to skip this stage, but the final relaxation is hugely important and one risks losing valuable prana by missing it. Yoga relaxation allows you to emerge refreshed and brings your body, mind, and spirit back into balance. It is great after a long day or while recovering from illness. Taking 20 minutes of conscious rest is enormously effective whenever you feel tired but need to keep working.

Many students gleefully exclaim "sleep!" when relaxation time, "yoga nidra," rolls around. Indeed, yoga nidra can be translated as yogic sleep, but remember that it is a conscious rest, requiring discipline. You practice being awake, yet free of body tension. After a strong session where you have really explored your boundaries, this active undoing comes easier. As you take a break from external movement, cease fidgeting, and lie perfectly still, the mind becomes acutely sensitive. While you progressively let go of tension in the muscles, bones, organs, even the brain, you remain aware of the internal sensations. Whenever your thoughts stray, bring them back to your body. As the senses quieten and attention is turned inward, there is a heightened awareness. Quietening the body and mind, drawing the senses inward, and accessing your inner peace are steps along the path to meditation.

Lying still with your eyes closed looks easy. But if you tend to move through life at a frenetic pace, never ceasing to stop and

*Above and opposite: Notice a feeling of expansion as your body settles into yoga relaxation.*

take stock, falling into quietness can seem difficult. Conscious relaxation is an exercise in yielding. So many of us cling tenaciously to objects, people, habits, or attitudes. The principal of detachment is fundamental to Eastern philosophies. While you remain strongly attached to things, their loss will inevitably cause suffering. If you observe yourself holding onto things and accumulating material possessions, use yoga relaxation to consciously practice letting go. Physically and mentally permit yourself to release that grip and be just you, nothing else, lying on the floor. As you actively undo, you let your defenses down and accept the sense of vulnerability inherent in allowing surrender.

Try making a fist with one hand and keeping it clenched for ten seconds. Now relax the fist and compare the feelings in the two hands. Most likely you'll feel more sensations in the hand that was clenched. As you seek to find the edge in each posture, you will be fully occupying both muscles and mind. Once the tension is released, a lingering awareness remains. The same principle applies in yoga relaxation. When you have extended your body to its limit, you'll notice how your awareness of internal sensations deepens because your mind has been completely engrossed in your practice. It will very easily let go into deep relaxation.

# GETTING COMFORTABLE FOR RELAXATION

Help yourself let go by becoming perfectly physically comfortable. Any of these modifications to the basic supine position may be helpful. *See* page 24 for how to make a "breathing bed." The Child Pose is useful whenever you need to relax during your practice or throughout your day.

## USING A PILLOW

Find the best position for your head by having a friend observe you as you lie on your back. Ideally, your chin and forehead will be at an equal height from the floor. If your chin is higher than your forehead, the back of the neck will tend to shorten. Many people don't need more than a thinly folded blanket to soften the floor for the head. However, if you find your chin juts up higher than your forehead when you are lying, make a pillow.

If the forehead is too high, the throat will feel constricted. Use a folded blanket to bring your chin and forehead level.

## MAKING A NECK PILLOW

Fold a blanket three times and roll it up about halfway. Wedge this securely under your neck, right up to shoulder level. Experiment with the amount of roll. Your neck should feel very snug with the roll supporting its natural curve. Usually the chin juts out a little, so fold the remaining flap down to cushion and lift the back of the head.

## SUPPORTING THE LOWER BACK

This support lets the lower back soften down closer to the floor, and those with lower back problems find it useful. Place large rolled cushions or a bolster under your knees, and do a small pelvic tilt to flatten the lower back toward the floor. Your lower back will still curve up away from the floor, but as you then lie and let go, you will feel it ease out and release a little. If you don't have any props, then bend your knees up, place your feet just wider than body width and lean the knees in together.

## COVER UP

When you relax deeply, your body temperature drops dramatically. It is impossible to let go completely when you are cold. Unless it is the height of summer, cover your whole body with a shawl or blanket.

## BALASANA—CHILD POSE

Sit on your heels with your knees together. Fold forward over your thighs. Rest your forehead to the floor and drape your arms around you. Close your eyes and let go of any tension. Enjoy the reassuring massage of the belly pressing down into the thighs with each inhalation. For high blood pressure, or if your buttocks stay high in the air and you feel like you are nosediving, rest the forehead on a pad of folded blankets. Alternatively, stack your fists one on top of the other to rest your forehead on.

# GUIDED RELAXATION IN SAVASANA CORPSE POSE

While this pose looks like the easiest of all the yoga asanas, it is actually one of the hardest to master. While the body lets go, the mind must stay alert, observing the relaxation process, before finally surrendering to rest. The final relaxation allows your body to settle and the effects of your Hatha yoga practice to consolidate. Spend about five minutes working through the body to exaggerate the tension in your muscles, section by section. This raises the level of awareness so you can better surrender to complete relaxation. A nice way to practice Savasana is to make a tape of these instructions, with plenty of pauses, or have a friend read them aloud.

**1.** Lie on your back in Savasana. Your legs are apart with feet rolling out to the sides. Your arms are just out from your sides. Have the backs of your hands on the floor so your fingers curl softly upward. Close your eyes so attention is drawn inward and you become sensitized to your inner environment.

**2.** Scrunch your toes and flex your feet. Next, spread out your toes and point the feet strongly. Then relax your feet.

**3.** Lift your right leg 2 in (5 cm) in the air. Briefly tense all the muscles in that leg and then release them, letting the leg fall to the floor. Do the same with the left leg.

**4.** Clench your buttocks for a few seconds so your hips rise up slightly. Release. Feel the heaviness of your lower body.

**5.** Tighten the muscles along the length of the spine and press the tips of your shoulders into the floor. Puff your chest up and tighten your abdominal muscles. Then exhale and relax the muscles, let the chest release down and allow the tension to flow out of the body.

## EXPLORE

As a general rule, for every 30 minutes of asana practice, practice at least five minutes of Savasana. For a 90-minute practice, allow 15 minutes of relaxation at the end.

But you don't need to practice any asanas to reward yourself with Savasana. Practice relaxation whenever you feel tired. Instead of taking a daytime nap, refresh with 20 minutes of Savasana.

**10.** Press the chin to the throat so you feel the back of the neck lengthening, then release it by softening all the neck muscles. So that you can commit to lying perfectly still for the next ten minutes, mentally check your position and adjust anything you need to. Just as during meditation, any outer movement will distract you from your inner world.

**11.** Become aware of the whole body being heavy and relaxed. Your body wants to be comfortable. It is in its natural state. The bones feel heavy. All the muscles are relaxed. The internal organs are free of tension. Even the tongue is relaxed. As the body releases and feels heavier, the breath lightens and feels more delicate. The brain surrenders any worries and is content, enjoying this peaceful and tranquil moment. Give permission for your emotional body to let go, too. While the body relaxes, the mind stays present, observing. Finally, completely stop trying to "do." Let go of any psychological effort at all. Now rest.

**6.** Lift one arm 2 in (5 cm) off the ground. Tighten all its muscles, make a fist with your hand, then stretch the fingers out. When you exhale let all the tension go so the arm drops back down on the floor. Repeat on the other side.

**12.** You will intuitively know when it's time to come out of the relaxation. Begin to move the fingers and toes as you focus back on the body. Take your arms overhead along the floor and stretch up through the body, enlivening everything from fingertips to toes. When you are ready, roll over onto your side and allow the eyes to open in their own time.

**7.** Lift the shoulders to the ears into a shrug and then release them back down and toward the hips.

**8.** Tighten all the facial muscles. Lose your inhibitions—no one is watching you! Clench your jaw muscles, squeeze the eyes tightly shut, and frown. Then widen everything out and apart. Open your eyes and roll the eyeballs back, open your mouth, and stick the tongue as far out toward the chin as you can. Finally, exhale with a sigh and relax the face. Feel all the skin on the face soften and any wrinkles smooth out.

**9.** This time without tensing, gently drop your right ear to the floor. Take a few long breaths and become aware of the stretch on the left side of the neck. Inhale the head to the center and drop the left ear to the floor for a few breaths before bringing the head to center again.

## EXPLORE

Your tongue is a huge muscle, attaching deep into the throat. There's much more of it than you can see when you stick it out. It usually sits touching the roof of the mouth. Instead, release it down so it floats in the center of the mouth. This relaxes the whole mouth, throat area and face. Observe whether this allows other more distant parts of the body to release, too.

# REVITALIZING RELAXATION

To make a "breathing bed," fold one to three blankets so they are 8 in (20 cm) wide and longer than your torso. Lie over them with your buttocks on the floor and legs a little apart. The more blankets you use, the more the chest will feel it is opening, so experiment with what feels best for you. Use another blanket as a pillow so that the head is higher than the chest. Take your legs apart and let your arms rest out to the sides.

Lie on your back and lift your head for a moment to look down your body to make sure you are perfectly symmetrical. After checking that you feel completely comfortable, begin to breathe deeply and rhythmically. As you inhale, visualize prana being drawn in through the nostrils down to your solar plexus. As you exhale it swirls around your center. With each inhalation, draw this pranic energy down to the solar plexus so that it spirals around filling up the whole torso. Each long, deep inhalation draws in more prana. While you are giving yourself the gift of vibrant energy, remember to keep the exhalations slow and steady. The full exhalation empties the lungs, allowing you to inhale this revitalizing force deeply and consciously.

From the center of the torso the spiral enlarges to cover the whole body. The outer part of the spiral reaches to circle over the head, fingertips, and toes. Let yourself become the breath. With this positive energy you become enthusiastic about life and your tasks. You gain the energy to fulfill them. Stay here as long as you need to.

When it is time to awaken, start moving your body and stretch a little. Feel so revitalized that the eyes blink open by themselves, as if powered by the energy within.

## WHITE LIGHT
To stay true to your inner self and protect yourself from being harmed or feeling drained by others, visualize yourself surrounded with glowing white light.

# HEALING VISUALIZATION

The use of color is a therapeutic branch on its own. White light gives strength of spirit, clarity and protection. Black, the absence of light, brings qualities of strength, power, evolution and transition. Yellow, the color of the intellect, is uplifting and joyful. Red fosters courage, warmth, and assertiveness. Orange is used for creativity, optimism, and tolerance. Sky blue is linked to sincerity, peace, honesty, and organizational abilities. Indigo promotes mental calmness and lessens attachment to material possessions. Violet fosters self-esteem and confidence, and dissolves the ego. Emerald green brings physical and emotional harmony and is recharging. Each chakra (*see* page 150) has a related color.

Choose a color to which to you feel intuitively drawn. As you lie quietly in Savasana, draw this color into any area of your body you would like to heal. With each inhalation, the color becomes clearer and brighter. It forms a dense core and, from there, begins to expand outward. In your mind's eye, visualize it expanding to fill the whole body: see it clearly filling your heart, a center for healing and unconditional love that keeps enlarging it. Take several minutes, allowing it to spill over to fill the whole body all the way down the legs to the toes, and all the way down the arms to the fingertips. Breathe this color up into your head. It fills your brain, the backs of your eyes, all the crevices behind the face. You happily accept the healing energy that your special color offers. You may like to send goodwill or healing to loved ones. Before you complete this exercise, mentally seal your color and its particular qualities in your body.

## CREATING A SANCTUARY

Think of a place where you know you can feel completely at ease. It could be a real place you have visited or seen or else an imaginary paradise—a special sanctuary where you feel completely safe, protected, and nurtured. It might be next to a still, deep pond, near the ocean, in a lush green forest or by a flickering fireplace in a wonderful home. Now, as you lie in Savasana, visualize yourself from above. From lying on the floor, visualize your body coming up to standing, and start on a pleasant trip toward your special place. Feel the sun on your skin and the breeze in your hair. Listen to the call of the birds and the other sounds around, like leaves in the gentle wind or a babbling brook. In time, you arrive at your special place and settle yourself down to sit in a meditative position. Visualize yourself sitting with eyes closed and a peaceful mind. Your sanctuary gives nourishment, and you are safe to relax completely. Continue to see yourself sitting quietly. Know that your sanctuary is always there when you need it. You just need to take the time to access it.

When it is time to come back, rouse yourself from sitting, and take the journey back to where you are lying, until you can see yourself on the floor again. Begin to tune in to the sounds around you. Feel the touch of the clothes on your skin, then roll over and sit up slowly.

## EXPLORE

Often mental anxiety around a health problem builds up. This creates more tension and pain. Practice directing calm, focused, accepting thoughts to that area. If only for a short time, separate yourself from your usual response to this challenge. Empty yourself of anxiety. Mentally send your breath to the area to release, soothe, and heal.

# BUILDING AWARENESS

The following exercises are good ways to reconnect with yourself at the start of a practice session.

## ABSORB YOURSELF IN YOUR BREATH

The stresses of day-to-day life can create different layers of breathing over our free, natural breath. This exercise will help you reconnect with your natural breath. Keep it simple. You are not aiming to go anywhere. You don't have to "do" anything. This is not a new technique, but rather a process of undoing. There is no need for effort, pushing or wanting. There is no search to attain the "perfect" breath. Instead, let it unravel. Often we are guided by our mental intelligence but, instead, let your instinctual natural physical intelligence take over as you unravel. Your body is what is breathing, not your mind. Your mind, relinquishing control, learns to move out of the way and becomes merely the accepting observer. Come back to this exercise regularly. Make sure that you allow at least 20 minutes for it.

**Above, below and opposite:** *Carry this breathing exercise over into the more vigorous asanas.*

Lie on your back with your knees bent and feet flat on the floor. Swivel your feet so your big toes are closer together than your inner heels, then lean your knees in together, so holding them in place is effortless. Have your arms out by your sides, palms facing down. Close your eyes. Give your full attention to your breathing. Can you feel where the breath originates? Observe which part of your body moves first as you breathe in. What happens next? Observe the sequence of your body's movement when you inhale. Feel what happens to the lower and upper abdomen. How do the ribcage and chest work? Can you feel anything happening at the back? What happens to the shoulders, throat, face, and nostrils? Does anything change at the pelvis?

Absorb yourself completely in your breath. You are your breath and your breath is you. It rises and falls with the rhythm of ocean waves. How do you accept your inhalation? How do you feel the expansion? Now turn your attention to the out breath. From where do you exhale? Which part of the body begins the movement? Where does your exhalation end? Are the movements in the torso as clearly demarcated as in your inhalation? Can you feel a consolidation of energy? Accept the support of the earth each time. Don't shrink, but let yourself sink.

Count the length of your in and out breaths. Which is longer? Does one come more easily to you? Become aware of the quality of your breath. Is it shallow or deep? How rhythmic does it feel? Does it feel smooth or coarse? Is it graceful and round, or are there some parts that feel jerky or jagged? Does it feel soothing?

Often we don't breathe out fully, but hurry on to the next inhalation. Take the time to follow the entire length of your exhalation. Stay with it. Patiently wait until it is finished before you take your next breath. It takes some time to release all the used air from the alveoli. There is no need to tighten any muscles to "squeeze" the last air out. Just be patient and let it keep on flowing. Whenever you feel you are trying too hard, release the effort.

Now become aware of the time at the end of the exhalation, before the next inhalation begins. There is a brief moment before your lungs call for air. Don't grab for the next breath. Sink into this natural pause and enjoy it. It is a moment of tranquillity, as still as a deep, calm pond. The exhalation disappears into it, and then the stillness gives birth to the inhalation. As you observe this stillness, you may find the pause lengthening naturally.

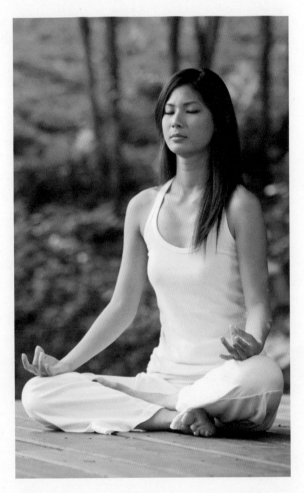

Now attune yourself to what happens at the top of the inhalation, before you feel the need to exhale. There is another pause, another precious moment. It is a full silence that you can relax into. As you let yourself sink into this moment, it will expand.

These pauses give rise to a breath in four parts: a releasing exhalation; a still pause; the gift of a new inhalation; and a pause. Become absorbed in a meditative way in each part of your breath. No two breaths are the same. Make friends with your breath and get to know each part intimately.

Before you roll over to sit up, take some time to observe the effects this exercise has had on your mind. You have learned a new skill to quieten the mind. You have developed your self-awareness, and practiced being absorbed in the present moment.

Have a friend read the instructions with plenty of pauses to allow you to explore.

# 1 CHEST OPENING EXERCISE

## AWARENESS OF THE BREATH

Channeling the breath into movement is centering and helps maintain a steady rhythmic breath.

1

**1.** Lie on your back with your knees bent up and your hands palms-down on the floor. To begin, exhale fully.

**2.** While you inhale, raise your arms up (2a) and overhead until the backs of your hands come to rest on or near the floor (2b). Energize your arms so that they extend and lift out of your shoulders to flow through a large arc.

2a

**3.** Exhale and raise your arms up to bring them back to the starting position. With eyes closed, continue moving between these two movements. Time the movement to follow your breath, not the other way around. Because you keep the flow of air in and out through the nostrils at a steady rate, your arm movements are also constant and graceful.

2b

**4.** Now become aware of how your torso moves in relation to the arm movements. As you inhale and raise the arms up, feel the natural life of the upper back as it lifts away from the floor. Rest with your arms overhead for several breaths. The upper back will ground more into the floor, and your chest will naturally open and promote a lovely full inhalation. Each time you exhale and bring your arms down, tune into the softening down which happens in the torso as it releases into the earth. Moving slowly, with awareness, bring your attention to your pelvis. Can you feel the gentle tilting backward and forward with each part of the breath? Take some more time, unhurriedly observing the movements of the body in response to the breath.

# BIRALASANA CAT POSE

This exercise brings awareness and flexibility to the entire length of the spine. The key to awareness is to move slowly. Practice patience and keep an inquiring mind.

**1.** Begin on all fours with your knees under your hips and your hands just forward of your shoulders.

**2.** Inhale and concave your back. Move your breastbone forward and up, and raise your tail bone up. Keep the back of your neck long as you gaze upward. Pressurize the palms evenly against the floor and avoid slumping into the shoulders.

**3.** As you exhale, round your back. Your upper back arches naturally in this way, so place particular awareness on the movement of the lower back as it follows this new curve upward as you tuck your pelvis under. Observe how your shoulder blades spread apart and the skin between them stretches. As you finish your exhalation, move your chin toward your breastbone.

**4.** Repeat ten more rounds, arching and rounding in time to your breath. Accentuate the curve so it is deeper each time.

# SUKHASANA FORWARD FOLD

## CROSS-LEGGED FORWARD FOLD

*Sukha* means "content" or "happy." Spending a few minutes letting yourself soften into this pose is a centering way to start your practice.

**1.** Sit in a simple cross-legged position. To work deeper into the hips, slide your heels away from each other so they rest under the knees. Then take the feet forward so the shins are in a horizontal line.

**2.** Become aware of the sitting bones in contact with the floor. This base will act as your anchor as you stretch forward. Place your fingertips on the floor just in front of your legs. Now lengthen the sides of the torso from hips to armpits. Use several breaths to let this releasing take place. When you feel ready, creep the hands away. Work with your breath as you take one or two minutes to slide the hands forward in stages. Only drop your forehead down to the floor if your front ribs come to lie on your legs. Then repeat with the legs crossed the other way.

## EXPLORE

Don't become mentally lazy. Stay aware. If you are performing the pose automatically, you might just stay at the point you initially reached. When you use longer holds in a pose, often you will find you can go much deeper and extend yourself to your new edge.

# 4 ROLL DOWNS

Working through this sequence will allow you to learn about how undoing, rather than active doing, can deepen a pose.

**1.** Stand in Tadasana (*see* page 36) with your feet hip-width apart. You are going to take several breaths to fold forward by rolling down the spine.

**2.** As you exhale, drop your head forward (2a). Feel how the shoulders want to follow. Release your knees so they bend slightly. On your next exhalation let the shoulders go and the upper back round more. Your arms hang down vertically, dangling passively out of their sockets (2b). Continue exhaling and rolling down the back in stages, leading with the head. Your knees will bend more the further you roll down. Take as many breaths as you need to release all the way down.

## EXPLORE

Repeat the same process, rolling down to each side in turn. Indulge by giving yourself plenty of time.

2a

**3.** Even though your legs are working, your upper body is dangling, hanging out of the hips. Bring a rag-doll quality to the upper body. Move your awareness to the shoulders and relax them fully so the arms hang loose. Relax the back of the neck so the crown of the head is the closest part of the head to the floor.

**4.** Take several rounds of breathing, observing the movements intrinsically related to the breath. As you inhale there is a lifting energy in the core of the body. If your knees are bent enough, a small lengthening occurs from pubic bone to throat. As you exhale, your ribs will fall closer to your thighs.

**5.** When it's time to come up, keep the knees bent and, over several breaths, roll up slowly through the spine, as if you are stacking each vertebra on top of the last. Exhale; release the arms down to the sides.

2b

3

# STANDING POSTURES

Within the standing postures you find side bends, backbends, forward
bends, twists, and balances. With the exception of the inverted positions,
they embody the effects of all the other groups of yoga postures.

Regular practice of the standing poses is a great start for all yogis.
They increase strength and flexibility in equal parts. As they extend
and integrate the whole body, they help correct imbalances of the
vertebral column. They develop grace, endurance, perseverance, and
concentration. They help you to feel energetic and enthusiastic.

As they involve the whole body, they warm you in
preparation for the other poses. As they are expansive poses,
you can more easily see the directions of energy extension as
the arms and legs extend out from the spine. You can use these
energies to give your poses a lightness. Over time, these poses
will even help to bring the spring back into flat feet.

In order to achieve anything in life, we need somewhere to
extend from. Standing postures let us develop roots. They allow
us to examine how we "stand on our own two feet" and how to
"stand our ground." They help us establish a firm base to ensure
the upper body is well supported. In standing poses we play off
stability with extension as we practice radiating outward from
this steady base.

## EXPLORE

Stay in your habitual standing position for long enough
without moving until the sensations begin to intensify.
Then take this feedback and see what you need to do
to realign and prevent the discomfort coming to those
points. Do this when you are sitting in your habitual way
in your favorite armchair, too.

## CAUTION

Avoid standing poses in acute cases of asthma, colitis,
nervous disorders, or cardiac problems. Don't jump in or
out of the poses if you are pregnant, menstruating, or if
you have back or knee injuries.

## EXPLORE

Sit on the floor and give your feet a little massage first. Do
small karate chops on the soles of the feet. Make loose fists
and do some light pounding. Rub your hands briskly over the
feet using the friction to build warmth. Now you might find it
easier to become aware of how your feet contact the earth.

## FROM THE GROUND UP

**1.** Have a look at your feet. How are the arches? Do they lift up or
do they collapse downward to produce flat feet or knock-knees?

How are your toes? Are they squashed together from
wearing tight shoes? Are they white with tension as
they cling to the ground? Ungrip the toes by lifting
them up and spreading them apart. Keeping them
stretched away, place them down on the floor.

**2.** Stand erect and feel where the heaviness comes
into the feet. Where is the weight centered? Is
there more weight placed on the balls of the feet,
or the heels? Is one foot taking more weight than
another? Rock back and forth to find your center.
Keeping the feet on the floor, transfer the weight
from left to right and back several times to home
in on the center of grounding. Lean in all directions
in a large circle. Then slowly reduce the size of the
circle until you find your centered point.

**3.** Mentally soften the soles of your feet.
Spread the skin. Let your breath come
into the feet. They widen and soften with
each exhalation. Visualize roots growing
downward. By earthing the feet, the rest of
the body is free to expand and lengthen.

# FROM THE PELVIS UP

**1. Anterior tilt.** Stand with hands on your hips, fingers pointing forward, so that your index fingers rest on top of the hip bones and press into the waist. Tilt your pelvis forward, just as if it were a basin and you were tipping water out of the front of it. Your fingers will point down and your thumbs will lift up. Feel how the curve in your lower back accentuates and your chest lifts a bit. This action makes the knees push back too.

**2. Posterior tilt.** Now tilt the pelvis the other way, as if you were pouring out water from the back. Your fingers will rise up and your thumbs move down. Your lower back curve will flatten and the fronts of your knees will move forward. The chest tends to slump, abdominal length shortens and shoulders roll forward. Feel how this affects your neck, too. If you are not sure, exaggerating the movements might help.

**3.** Come back to the center, so your pelvis is not tipped forward or back, but centered. Take time to feel how it is mentally, comparing it to your normal way of standing.

By taking time to move in between the anterior and posterior pelvic tilt positions, you will become familiar with the trickle-on effects of them on the rest of your body. A truly centered pelvis would actually be too unstable to carry us well, so people tend to have a pelvis tilted either one way or the other. Ideally, this position would be just off center, rather than strongly so. Still standing, find a more centered position for your pelvis. Observe how your body feels when comparing it to your normal way of carrying yourself. Slowly move around the room like this, exploring new possibilities for carriage and movement.

# ELONGATING THE CURVES OF THE SPINE

**1.** Stand with your back to a wall or doorframe. Take your feet about 1 ft (30 cm) away from the wall, and a little bit apart, with the outside edges of the feet parallel. Lean against the wall so your body contacts the wall at the sacrum and the thoracic curve. The small of the back (lumbar region) will arch away from the wall. How easily the back of your head comes to the wall depends on the curves of your spine. If your upper back is very flat, your throat will feel constricted. If your upper back is very rounded, it will be more difficult to bring your head comfortably to the wall. If your chin juts out and the back of the neck shortens, find a midway position for the head. Gently bring your floating ribs down, so they don't jut out. Don't bend your knees. Bring the tops of the thighs back slightly so the front of the groin opens.

**2.** The spine is most effectively lengthened by undoing, rather than doing. Take plenty of time to release so the spine can elongate upward. If you actively work the muscles that run along the spine, then they will contract and actually shorten the vertebral column. Likewise, there is no need to raise the shoulders up to grow taller. Instead, let go with each exhalation. Let your tail bone be heavy so it eases down toward the floor. Keep your weight well grounded through your feet. As you continue to lengthen, feel the very small movements that ripple along the spine in connection with the breath. Are there any areas of your spine that feel blocked? Concentrate on softening the tight spots. When you move away from the wall, walk softly around the room, feeling the effects of this exercise.

# TADASANA Mountain Pose

5

This pose connects you to both earth and sky. It is a wonderful exercise in centering and being able to respond to situations from a solid base. Begin and end each of the standing poses with this centered position. Use it as a chance to hear your body's feedback to what happened in the last pose. Although you appear steady as a mountain, you are not as hard as a rock in this pose. Externally your mountain is still, but bring it alive from the inside where it feels dynamic and alive, responding to every breath. Practice Tadasana whenever possible throughout the day.

**1.** Stand with your feet a little less than hip-width apart, with the outside edges of your feet parallel. Follow the instructions for softening the feet on page 34. While your feet ground downward, move your awareness to your legs and get a sense of extending up toward the sky starting at the ankle joints. Let your pelvis be in a neutral position (*see* previous page). The spine, supported by the pelvis, is freed to lengthen upward. It is perfectly possible to stand erect and be relaxed at the same time. Exhale tension out of the spine so it is released to grow taller. Feel your arms dangling from the shoulder sockets. Let them hang, and completely let go. As your shoulders soften down, the neck and head float and rise up out of them. Release the mouth, tongue, and jaw. Observe whether this allows other more distant parts of the body to release, too. Bring a sense of weightlessness to the head. Visualize it as a helium-filled balloon on the end of a stick, your spine. Mentally sweep over your body to see where the heaviness is.

**2.** Check in with your breathing. Release the diaphragm muscle. Take slow, deep, steady breaths. Feel the ripple-like effect of each breath on the spine. Quite different from an upward movement induced by muscle tension, feel the lifting energy with each inhalation. Your body has its own innate intelligence. Be curious! Follow your breath to feel where it lets your body open and expand. Explore any subtle effects that your exhalation has on it.

# PRASARITA PADOTTANASANA
## WIDE LEG STRETCH

In asanas the arms and legs often act as levers to work the spine. But make sure they work with the rest of your body and breath, not forcefully overriding them.

**1.** From Tadasana, step your feet wide apart. Have your toes facing straight ahead and the outside edges of the feet parallel. Bring your hands to your hips. With the heels heavy on the floor, let the tail bone drop down to the earth. This helps make space between the vertebrae of the lower back and protects them from compressing. Firm the front of the thigh muscles, open the groin and expand the breastbone up to the sky as you look up and back. Hold for several breaths.

## EXPLORE

Interlace your fingers behind your back and take your arms overhead. Firm your front thigh muscles as your thumbs move toward the floor.

**2.** On an exhalation, fold forward. If possible, position both palms on the floor, shoulder-width apart, upper arms parallel. If you are still developing your hamstring flexibility, bend your knees if necessary to bring your fingertips to the floor. Unhunch shoulders by sliding the shoulder blades up toward the hips. Walk the hands back as they lever you deeper into a forward bend. When it is time to come up, bring your hands back onto your hips. Firm the thigh and abdominal muscles and inhale to come up.

# VIRABHADRASANA I Warrior I

This all-involving pose works the arms and legs, strengthens the back, and opens the chest.

**1.** Stand with your legs about 4 ft (1.2 m) apart. Turn your whole right leg and foot deeply inward 60 degrees. Turn your left leg and foot out 90 degrees and swivel your whole upper body so it faces over your left leg. Open the right groin by letting your left hip move forward to align with the right. If this is difficult, turn the back leg and foot in deeper. An easier alternative is to have the feet parallel and lift up the back heel off the floor (*see* alternative opposite).

**2.** Bend your left knee to a 90-degree angle. Keep your back leg straight by pressing the back heel away to open the back of the knee.

**3.** Take your arms out to the sides, turn the palms up and raise the arms overhead to join the palms. Gaze at your thumbs. Stretch up from the hips to the fingertips. As you breathe deeply, feel the stretch of skin on the chest and abdomen. Stay for ten breaths, and maintain perfect awareness as you come out of the pose and move to the right side.

## EXPLORE

In these wide-stance poses, have your feet lined up so the heel of the front foot bisects the center of the back foot. You can even draw a line along the center of your mat.

# ALTERNATIVE: HEEL LIFTED

An easier alternative for beginners is to have the feet parallel and lift up the back heel off the floor. If you have trouble balancing, step the front foot a little to the side. Sometimes people unconsciously hunch their shoulders when attempting to press their palms together. Until your shoulder flexibility develops, take your palms apart and arms parallel and check if this releases it. If you still feel "bad" shoulder tension, then lower your arms 10 or 20 degrees forward, with attention to spreading the shoulder blades well apart.

# VIRABHADRASANA II WARRIOR II

8

As if you were aiming a bow and arrow at your target, maintain a perfect mental focus over your middle finger. Strong legs give self-reliance and independence and the raised head, fearlessness.

**1.** From Tadasana take the feet wide apart, so that when your arms are stretched out, your ankles will be underneath them. Rotating from the top of the thigh, turn the right leg and foot inward 15 degrees. Turn the left leg and foot out 90 degrees. This tends to alter the position of the hips. Bring your hands onto your hips to help you compare them. If your right hip is higher and more forward than the left hip, adjust them so they are in line.

2

**2.** Bend your left knee to a 90-degree angle, not more. If your knee is positioned in front of your ankle, then you need to widen your stance. As the toes of your left foot are facing out to the side, your knee should be obscuring your view of all except your big toe. Look down the front of your torso to check that the ribs on both sides are even.

## EXPLORE

To protect your knees, they must be
facing the same direction as the toes of
their respective feet.

3

**3.** Rotate your upper arms outward so the palms turn out.
Then raise your arms until they are parallel with the floor.
Finally, rotate just the forearms so the palms face down to the
floor—the creases of your elbows will remain facing upward.
Drop your shoulders down. Become aware of two lines of energy
radiating from your spine out to your fingertips. Use this feeling
to help keep your arms parallel to the floor. Turn your head to
gaze at your left index finger. Take ten slow, steady breaths before
repeating on the right side.

# TRIKONASANA
## TRIANGLE POSE

9

This pose has five rays of energy: two arms stretching away, two legs stretching out and down, and a fifth line running from the tail bone as it extends toward the crown of the head.

1

**1.** From Tadasana, jump or step the feet 4–4$^1$/$_2$ ft (1.2–1.4 m) apart. Turning from the thighs, rotate the right foot inward 15 degrees and turn the left foot out 90 degrees. Level off your hips. If your legs are not working fully, your kneecaps will slump down and inward, so activate your thigh muscles to ensure the kneecaps track over the toes. Take your left hand near your knee. This is a strong side stretch so the body needs to be on one plane. Your hip bones, shoulders, and hands should be along the same line as your feet. To open the chest and keep your single-plane alignment, wrap the other arm around the back to wedge the hand by the inner thigh, or else take hold of the back of your pants. Assist this action by bending the front knee.

**2.** Draw your left sitting bone down toward your right inner heel so your hips move to the right. As you do this, straighten your left leg and slide the left hand down the leg or possibly to the floor as pictured. If you find your shoulders have come forward of your feet, and your buttocks have moved back, adjust your alignment by bringing your left hand higher up your leg. Roll your right shoulder back and enjoy the openness in the chest for several breaths before eventually releasing your right arm to vertical. Stretch out well from abdomen to feet, and from shoulders toward each hand. Intensify the line of energy from tail bone to crown of the head by sliding the shoulder blades away from the ears to keep the back of the neck long. Tuck the chin slightly in, turn the head and gaze at the right thumb.

Stay for five to ten breaths, then repeat on the right side.

2

## EXPLORE

Sit on the floor with your legs in front of you. When your thighs are relaxed, you will be able to move your kneecap from side to side. Activate your thigh muscles to straighten the legs and raise your heels off the ground. Now you won't be able to move the kneecap from side to side. Use this activation of the thighs, not forced or locked, but firm and aware, in Trikonasana.

# UTTANASANA INTENSE FORWARD STRETCH

If you suffer from hypertension, keep the trunk parallel to the floor and place your hands on a chair or table. Begin working through this sequence with Roll Downs (*see* page 32).

## USING A WALL

**1.** To maintain length in the front of the torso, practice using the wall. Stand with your feet apart and about 1 ft (30 cm) away from the wall. Lean your buttocks to the wall so your sitting bones touch it. Hold your elbows and take the arms overhead. Bend the knees and extend the torso up so the top of the breastbone, moves away from the pubic bone. With knees strongly bent, reach your torso forward. Stretch as far out with the elbows as possible. Fold over your legs and let your upper body hang for ten breaths or more. With each inhalation the torso can lengthen more, and with each exhalation the crease at the top of the thighs can deepen. If you can't work in a relaxed fashion into this position, bend the knees more or walk the feet further away from the wall. Come up on an inhalation.

**2.** Move away from the wall. Bring your hands onto your hips, inhale, lift your breastbone and look up. Exhale, hinge at the hips to reach forward so the crown of the head moves in as big an arc as possible. Imagine your hip sockets and pelvis rolling forward over your thigh bones, which stay vertical.

1

2

3

**3.** With your knees bent or straight, grasp your legs or ankles, or loop your big toes with finger and thumb. Increase the stretch by flattening out the back and stretching your sternum forward. Angle your sitting bones toward the sky, lengthen the back of your waist. Tilt your pelvis forward as if aiming to press your navel to your thighs—you will feel the stretch in the back of your thighs intensify.

4

**4.** Then exhale and fold forward to hold the pose. If your knees are bent, use each exhalation to work the legs straighter. If your legs are straight, firm the front thigh muscles and bring your hips forward to bring the hip joints directly over your ankles.

Check that your face is relaxed. Free the upper lip so your cheeks feel like they are dropping down toward the floor. If you have forgotten to breathe, check whether the pose is too strong for you and ease back until you free the breath.

# EXPLORE

Working the feet correctly in the standing poses helps to retrain flat feet over time. If you have flat feet, lift your toes up to work the arches in the standing postures. Alternatively, anchor the inner heel and mound of the big toe and, without rolling the ankles out, lift your arches like rainbows.

# 11 PAVRITTA TRIKONASANA
## REVOLVED TRIANGLE POSE

This advanced pose combines balance, twisting, and forward bending. In the wide-stance poses, the further apart the feet are, the greater the spinal extension, but the more difficult it becomes to balance.

**1.** Stand with your feet 3–4 ft (1–1.2 m) apart. Turn your left foot and leg well inward to about 60 degrees and turn the right foot out 90 degrees. Bring your left hip forward so it's level with the right hip. Stretch your left arm up in the air and take several breaths, getting a sense of the full extension all the way from the left ankle to the left hand.

## EXPLORE

Looking down to the floor makes it easier to balance while
you increase the twist in the trunk. Take several breaths gazing
at the floor to allow a deeper rotation. Finally, turn the head
to look forward and slowly up to the top thumb.

**2.** On an exhalation, reach the left arm and torso forward and
down to bring the left hand to cup the floor by the right little toe.
If the hand doesn't reach, place the hand on the seat of a chair or
on a stack of books. With both feet and the left hand anchored,
stretch the right hip back to help the extension of the spine out
of the hips. Rotate the torso well to the right so the navel and
heart open up to the sky. Take the right arm
straight up into the air and gaze
up at your right thumb.

# FORWARD BENDS

Sometimes in our outward-looking lives, we ignore messages from inside.
Folding into ourselves quietens the mind and encourages a meditative mindset.
Forward bends foster the ability to listen to our intuitive self, to our heart.

Gravity often helps us fold forward; we can go deeper into the pose by yielding rather than forcing. From the seated position, we don't even have to be concerned with balancing, and can take energy and support from the earth. The forward bends are a little like the foetal position and have nurturing qualities for when we need to feel protected.

As you fold in half from your hips, your head comes closer to your feet. The two extremes of the body come together and help you find your center. Life is full of dualities. Rather than operating from one end of the spectrum, you can find a better balance: moderation and the middle path in our world view and way of living.

By increasing pressure on the organs of the abdomen, forward bends are particularly beneficial to the digestive system. As the pelvis houses nerve ganglions of the parasympathetic nervous system, they also help balance the nervous systems. The parasympathetic nervous system directs our "rest and restore" response. Forward bends are helpful for those with active, busy (sympathetic nervous system dominant) lives, and for anyone who seeks healing and better health.

Forward bends can be done in a very active way, with strong breathing to help release deeper into the postures. Alternatively, when you are experiencing menstrual discomfort, feel fatigued, or need to revive, they can be done softly, and made more restorative using a chair or a bolster. Rest the forehead on a chair seat covered by a soft blanket. If you are more flexible, use a bolster.

Don't overdo the forward bends if you suffer from severe depression. Focus on backbends instead. Those suffering hypertension do best to keep their head above their heart. Forward bends maintain integrity of the spine, but proceed cautiously if you have back pain. If a weakness exists or if you are recovering from an injury, it is always best to build your practice in a slow and steady way. If you suffer from disk problems, that section of the spine needs to be kept concave and should not be bent forward until it is ready. Work with a teacher to implement forward bends into your practice bit by bit as your back strengthens. Allow 24 hours after the practice for your body to give you its feedback.

*Left and oppposite:*
*Develop patience and the ability to stay longer in the forward bends.*

# ABOUT ALIGNMENT
## DISCOVERING THE ACTION OF THE PELVIS AND HIPS

It's worthwhile investing some time to discover how to get the most benefit out of forward bends.

**1.** Sit erect in your chair and place your hands on your waist. Lower your chin to your chest, then bring your head down toward your thighs. You will feel the stretch mostly along the sides of the spine. Observe how your shoulders hunch and your back rounds. You might also notice that it's difficult to take deep breaths.

**2.** Sit up straight again and lower your hands from your waist to your hips. Inhale, expand the chest, lengthen your spine up, and gaze forward. As you exhale, fold forward, leading with the chest. With this movement you hinge from the hips. Compared with the last exercise, the spine is kept relatively straight (which protects the intervertebral disks) and you will feel the stretch more in the hips and back thighs than in the spine. This is the movement required by the yoga forward bends. Practice these two variations a couple more times so you are clear in your mind about the difference. Imprint the memory of this second exercise in your body so you can bring it alive during every yoga forward bend that you will encounter in the future.

**3.** It helps if we understand where we place our seat when sitting erect. The two sitting bones (ischial tuberosities) act as little anchors to the earth. As you sit on the floor, reach under your buttocks and move your buttock flesh away, in a direction 45 degrees back and out to the side, to help your sitting bones to contact the ground.

4

**4.** If you have a lack of flexibility in the hamstrings, you will tend to sit on the back edge of your sitting bones. The pelvis will be tilted backward, as the tight hamstrings pull around the corner on the lower back and flatten the normal lumbar curve. Your stomach muscles have to work hard to keep you upright, so sitting in this position won't be comfortable. It also creates a tendency to concave the chest. A forward bend born from this position will inevitably be a forward bend from the waist, instead of the hips. Apart from closing the chest to deep breathing, by pressurizing the fronts of the intervertebral disks, the spine will not maintain a healthy alignment. The ideal starting position will be sitting right on the center of the sitting bones so that as you fold your body forward, you will roll forward to perch more on the front edge of your sitting bones.

**5.** While sitting on the floor, touch your lower back. If your lower back still flattens or rounds out instead of keeping its usual inward curve, then your pelvis will be tilting backward. As you need to move from sitting on the back edge of the sitting bones to being on their center, modify your starting position. Lift your seat with folded blankets, and/or bend your knees. Use one or both of these adjustments in your forward bends for as many months as it takes for your body to loosen.

5

**6.** It is better to do a smaller-looking forward bend with correct alignment than a seemingly deeper forward bend, which at worst may be injurious and at best doesn't help release the areas that are chronically tight. Keep the length in the spine by extending the tail bone and crown of the head away from each other. As you fold forward, stretch your tail bone back and away from the crown of the head. Moving the sitting bones back increases the stretch in the hamstrings.

**7.** As you fold forward, visualize your thigh bones staying still. It is actually the sockets of the hip joints that can rotate around the heads of the thigh bones to tilt the pelvis forward. When you can achieve this, the concavity in the lumbar spine will remain for the first part of the forward bend. Test this by placing your hand on your lower back to feel if you have the same curve during the first part of the forward bend. Toward the end of your stretch forward, you will feel the shape of the lumbar spine change and begin to curve outward.

**8.** Let go of your desire to reach your forehead to your knees. Instead, first aim the navel to the thighs. As you hinge more at the hips, your chest will come closer to your knees, and only after this will the nose come toward the shins.

# DANDASANA STAFF POSE

## 12

Dandasana is the base from which we fold forward into many forward bends.

### EXPLORE

Because this position is outwardly simpler than many others, it provides a good opportunity to take your attention inward. Take slow, conscious breaths. In this position it is possible to focus not only on the forward and sideward expansion of the torso, but also on the expansion of the back of the torso as you inhale and the lungs fill with air.

Sit with your legs straight out in front. If it is hard to sit with the back erect in this pose, and you tip back, sit on one or two folded blankets. Place your fingertips or palms on the floor by the buttocks. Roll the thigh bones inward so the inner thighs come together. Have the fronts of the kneecaps and the toes pointing straight upward. Straighten the knees so the backs of the knees are stretched. Let the arms lengthen. Let the breastbone float up, but not at the cost of shortening the back. Ensure your chin is not jutting out, but is kept parallel to the floor. Imagine your head floating on the top of your spine like a helium balloon on the top of a stick. Lighten your thoughts!

# VIRASANA Hero Pose

Although children sit like this quite naturally, older, stiffer bodies can find this pose uncomfortable. Use props as necessary while you regain your flexibility.

**1.** Kneel on the floor with your knees together and feet wide apart. As you sit down between your feet, use your fingers to "iron" your calf muscles out to the sides and down toward the heels.

2

**2.** Place your hands on the soles of your upturned feet. Lift up from your pubic bone to the notch of the throat. Lift up on the back of the body too, from the tail bone to the crown of the head.

3

**3.** If your buttocks don't come down to the floor, then create as much height as you need to be comfortable but still with a degree of challenge. Use bolsters, cushions, or folded blankets as a prop, or an old telephone directory; each time you practice, tear out a few pages so that over time you are able to sit comfortably on the floor.

**4.** If you experience knee pain, place a canvas belt or thin folded scarf deeply in the crease of the knees as they bend.

**5.** If this position gives pain on the tops of the feet, place some cushioning underneath the fronts of the ankles.

## EXPLORE

Forward bend from this pose. Lean forward onto your hands or, if you are more flexible, stretch the arms all the way forward with fingers interlaced.

# TRIANGA MUKHAIKAPADA PASCHIMOTTANASANA

## THREE-LIMBED FORWARD BEND

If forward-bending Virasana is too much of a challenge for now, warm yourself up by practicing one leg at a time.

**1.** From Dandasana, bend your right leg back to bring the foot to the floor next to the buttocks. As in Virasana, "iron" your calf flesh out to the right. As you will tend to tilt to the left, mentally let your right sitting bone be heavy so that you stay balanced and don't tip over.

2

**2.** Sometimes it is useful to use a flowing movement to ease into a pose. On an inhalation, reach your arms up to the sky and then fold forward as you exhale. On the next inhalation, reach the arms out and up once more, and flow forward as you exhale. After five cycles, hold the forward bend for five to ten long breaths. Repeat on side two.

## ALTERNATIVE

To align the spine and better balance the hips, place a support under one buttock.

## EXPLORE

Try this way of working in some poses. If you hold a pose for 15 breaths, use the first five to adjust and deepen the posture. For the remaining ten breaths, remain steady at a still point. At this point you still the fluctuations of the body, and are moving neither from nor toward any point. Be receptive to your observations.

## PASCHIMOTTANASANA

This is the classic Paschimottanasana. Sit in Dandasana. Keep your knees and toes pointing to the sky. Lengthen from the tail bone to the crown of the head. After several breaths "growing" the spine, inhale and raise the arms overhead, then exhale the arms and torso forward. Remember the feeling from the first exercise—keep the chest open and the breath free. Depending on your flexibility, hold one wrist around the feet, hook your toes, grasp the sides of your feet or ankles, or loop a belt around the balls of the feet. Take long, slow breaths for 10 to 15 rounds.

# 15 ARDHA BADDHA PADMA PASCHIMOTTANASANA

## BOUND HALF-LOTUS FORWARD FOLD

Due to the position of the arms in this hip-opening stretch, it is difficult to "cheat" by rounding the shoulders. Warming up the hip will help prevent knee problems and assist the movement of the knee toward the earth. Apart from this warm-up, you can practice the ankle to knee pose (see page 64).

1

**1** Warm up the hip by cradling your right leg. If cradling is difficult, then hold the knee and foot in both hands and push them slightly together. Slowly move the leg back and forth as you would rock a baby. Keep your right foot flexed as you slowly move the knee beyond the armpit. If you find this movement easy, then lift the right foot up higher.

**2** Take the bent leg to the floor and out to the side. Hold the top of the foot, and slide it onto the other thigh until the ankle is resting on the thigh—if you only bring the top of the foot to the thigh, the ligaments of the outside of the foot risk being overstretched. Reach around with your right hand and take hold of the foot.

3

**3** Stretch forward and take your right hand to the right foot, ankle, or shin. Release your left knee down to the floor. Hold for five to ten breaths. Repeat on the other side.

## ALTERNATIVE
If you can't reach, loop a belt around your shin and hold both ends with your left hand.

## EXPLORE
Remind yourself that it is irrelevant how far you look like you go in a pose. The important thing is to reach the point where you can learn and change. Measure your posture not by how flexible you are, but by how steady your breath is.

# UPAVISTA KONASANA

## SEATED WIDE-ANGLE POSE SEQUENCE

Have patience as you hold this pose.
Wait for the body to let you in.

**1.** Sit with your legs out to the sides at about a 90-degree angle. In this pose it is easy to let the kneecaps roll backward or forward, so check that your kneecaps and toes point straight up. Place your right hand, palm up, on your right thigh. Inhale and raise your left arm up, then curve over to the right so the sides of your body curve out like a rainbow. Keep your left shoulder on the same plane as your right, not in front of it. "Puff" out the left side ribs and draw the right side ribs into the body. Imagine the spaces between the left sides of each vertebra stretching apart. Slide your right hand down your leg. Hold for at least five breaths.

2

**2.** Now twist your torso toward the floor as you lower your left shoulder and arm. Bring the left hand near the right to stretch over your right leg. Turn the toes back and extend through both heels. Anchor down through the left sitting bone. Hold for five to ten breaths.

**3.** Now you have arrived at Upavista Konasana. Walk the hands in a wide arc toward the center. Ease back a little so you can tune into the sensation of the trunk lifting out of the hips. Slide the hands forward as you release in stages over about a minute.

**4.** When you have completed this sequence on both sides, support under your knees with your hands as you bring your legs together for Dandasana.

3

## CAUTION
You should not experience inner knee pain in this pose. If you do, make sure you are working the legs by stretching out through the heels, and firming the thigh muscles to the bone. Narrow the distance between the legs and ease off on the stretch.

# 17 BADDHA KONASANA

## COBBLER'S POSE

Translated from Sanskrit as "Bound Angle Pose," this position is also called "Cobbler's Pose" because it is the position in which shoemakers in India sit to work.

1

**1.** Raise your seat with a support like a cushion and bring the soles of your feet together. Draw your heels up close toward you. Use the pressure of your hands on the floor behind you to tilt the pelvis forward. As you do so, let the breastbone float up. These two movements will begin the opening along the inner thighs and groin. With the support of your hands behind you, move the knees away from each other, back and down to the floor. If your hips are tight, this may be as far as you go in this pose for today.

2

**2**. If your pelvis tips forward easily, you can dispense with the cushion before bending your elbows into the calves and bind the feet with your hands. Inhale and create the sensation of the torso lifting out of the pelvis. Exhale and deepen the fold. On each inhalation, lengthen from pubic bone to throat; each exhalation is an opportunity to move out and down. Rather than butterflying the knees up and down, work with the breath to soften the tight areas. Breathe evenly for five to ten rounds.

## EXPLORE

Sit on the floor in this position whenever possible. Lean back against the sofa in Cobbler's Pose while you watch television.

# SUPTA PADANGUSTASANA

## RECLINING BIG TOE POSE

This pose keeps the back stable and helps prevent it overstretching by moving the stretch more into the hamstrings. For those who are recovering from a herniated disk, this pose is a safe forward bend to practice on the road to recovery.

**1.** Lie on your back with your knees bent up. Lift your right leg up and loop a belt around the ball of the foot. Straighten the leg. As you inhale, imagine a line of energy extending from right buttock to right heel. As you exhale, yield a little to stretch the back of the leg more.

**2.** Release tension in the shoulders. Check the chin is not jutting up in the air—if it is, slide the back of the head away to bring it down.

**3.** If you are ready to move on to stage two, straighten the left leg along the floor and stretch out through both heels. As your flexibility grows, your leg will form an acute angle with your torso. Then you will be able to work the pose by holding the big toe of the raised foot. Until this comes, use the belt. After one to two minutes in this position, inhale and curl your head and upper back off the floor to bring your nose to your knee. Walk your hands higher up the belt. Hold for seven breaths and when you exhale down, keep the hands at that height and, seemingly miraculously, your body may be able to accept the increased stretch.

**4.** For this next stage, it is important to keep the left leg straight as it acts as your anchor. In the beginning, use your left hand to press down on the top of your left thigh. Holding the belt or side of your foot, take your right leg out to the side. Although you may not get that high this practice, aim to take your toes to the floor at shoulder level. Do this movement slowly so you don't lose the grounding force of the left upper thigh and left heel. If you start to tip, come back up and press both sides of the sacrum down to the floor before lowering down again.
Hold for five to ten breaths.

4

5

**5.** Come back to center and hold your big toe, or both ends of the belt, in your left hand. Turn your toes inward and anchor down the sacrum on the right side. It helps to press down with your thumb at the root of the thigh. Take the leg over to the left and hold for five to ten breaths. Come back to stretching through the center before lowering the leg down to repeat on the second side.

# EXPLORE

Before you do this hip-releasing sequence, lie flat and look at your feet. Your toes will be turned out—measure how much the toes of each foot are turned out, checking the difference between sides. This sequence releases the hips. Visually measure it again after each side.

# 19 GOMUKHASANA Cow Face Pose

Sometimes the poses we find most difficult are the very ones we can benefit most from practicing.

## EXPLORE

If this pose comes easily to you, lower the arms and lean forward onto the hands. Then try bringing your heels forward so they are on the same transverse plane as your buttocks. Now place your hands on the floor in front of you and lean forward to deepen the stretch.

**1.** Warm the hips up first by sitting cross-legged. Take the left ankle and place it on the top of the right knee. Make sure it is the ankle, not the outer part of the top of the foot, so that the ligaments in that area are not stretched too much. If your top shin is more or less parallel to the floor, then you can place your hands on the floor in front and stretch forward. Otherwise, breathe into the hips from an upright position to help loosen them. Repeat on the other side. Another useful warm-up is cradling the leg (*see* page 56).

1

**2.** Kneel, then cross your left knee over your right knee. As you sit back in the space between your feet, let your right knee stay on the floor. Your left knee will lift and ideally sit neatly on top of the right. However, if you are less flexible it may come up in midair. Raise your seat with folded blankets if you would like to make it easier.

**3.** Take your right arm straight up in the air. Rotating from the shoulder, turn the little finger to the front. Extend the distance from right hip to fingertips. Then bend the elbow to lower your forearm behind you. Hold the elbow with your left hand and take several breaths as you ease your right hand further down your back. When your right shoulder has grown accustomed to the stretch, release your left arm down. From the left shoulder, rotate the arm so your thumb turns inward, then back. Bend the arm to grasp your hands together. Move the back of the head back—don't let the head tilt down to one side. As you sit tall and breathe 10 to 15 breaths, be aware of the expansion of the right side ribs in this position. Repeat on the other side.

3

## ALTERNATIVE

For tight shoulders, grasp a soft belt and use time and the breath to help you inch your hands together.

# AFTER FORWARD FOLDING

20

These stretches act as counter-poses after some intense forward bending.

## Z POSE

Kneel on a cushioned surface if you like. Stretch the arms forward, parallel to the floor. Tuck the tail bone under, open the groin, and lean back to form a "Z" shape.

## SAVASANA VARIATION

**Corpse Pose Variation**

Resting in Corpse Pose with the arms overhead brings a slight backbend to balance the body.

## PURVOTTANASANA

**Stretch on the East Side of the Body**

From Dandasana, lean back, point the toes, lift your hips high, and fully expand your chest.

## PURVOTTANASANA

**Easier Version**

Begin with bent knees, lift the hips and chest up, then stretch the chin away.

# BACKBENDS

Like the forward bends, the backbends help keep the spine supple and well aligned to promote good functioning of the nerves, which innervate the rest of the body.

## BACKBENDS

Sit erect, take a deep inhalation, look up, and notice how the spine seems to lengthen, grow and extend. Congratulations! You have begun a lovely backbend!

If you think of what you do every day, you will notice that many of your activities involve bending forward. Sitting at a desk to work, at a table to eat, driving, doing housework, or gardening all tend to shorten the front of the body. Even the habit of looking at the ground while walking can put a stoop in good posture. Backbends realign the spine, counteract rounded shoulders, and help us move with poise and grace.

Backbends are exciting, energy-raising and warming. Repeat any active backbend a few times in a cold room and you will soon feel the heat created. Backbends keep the spine young and supple. They activate the abdominal region and stimulate blood supply to the kidneys, reproductive system, and digestive organs.

The vertebral column houses the main subtle energy pathway, the Sushumna Nadi. Backbends help shunt energy up the spine and through the chakras—the centers of energy—along the way. Working especially from the second to fifth chakras, energy blockages are released and stagnant areas invigorated.

You need courage, determination, and willpower to hold strong backbends, the very same qualities that are linked to the third chakra at the solar plexus. Backbends build character, strength, and confidence, which is what people mean when they refer to someone who "has backbone." You can develop "backbone" to deal with change and pressure in other parts of your life as you explore your full range of flexibility. Integrity of the spine can help create integrity of the mind. It is hard to think about anything else when you are breathing strongly in a strong backbend, so, by making the mind and body alert, backbends help combat depression and lethargy.

When we feel unsafe we instinctively fold in on ourselves. Bending backward counteracts this curling up and brings us out of our shelter. Lengthening and opening along the belly exposes our visceral organs, giving us practice in dealing with vulnerability. Backbends are like exploring uncharted territory. They allow us to practice spreading awareness to unfamiliar parts of the body. We never see our backs directly, needing instead to twist around to catch a reflection in a mirror. Bending backward is leaning into new terrain, requiring us to conquer the fear of the unknown.

In opening the heart center, backbends are enormously uplifting. The chest lifts and widens to encourage better breathing and full expansion of the lungs. Expanding the heart center uncramps, rejuvenates and welcomes joyful vitality into your life.

Always warm up with some standing postures before beginning backbends. To really feel your backbends develop, repeat the pose three times. The body does tend to feel the effects of holding backbends, so follow with some of the counter-poses on pages 82–83.

Those suffering from hypertension or heart trouble should work with an experienced teacher. Avoid strong backbends during menstruation, pregnancy, and for eight weeks after giving birth. Those with a herniated disk, lumbar injury, peptic, or duodenal hernia, or who have recently had surgery can practice mild backbends. If weakness of the back or discomfort is present, build up your practice slowly and progressively.

*Above and opposite: You must protect the vulnerable lower back and neck, making these parts stronger, and bringing awareness to them.*

# ABOUT ALIGNMENT
## SPECIAL PREPARATIONS FOR BETTER BACKBENDS

Stretch the legs and trunk and open the shoulders before backbending.
Warm up the body with these exercises and your backbending will
come more easily.

### NECK EXTENSION

Elongating the neck teaches you how to extend it in backbends
without compressing the cervical spine.

**1.** Sit on your heels and drop your head
back. Mentally visit your neck and observe
how that feels. Notice how far back your
gaze arrives.

**2.** Now interlace your fingers at the base
of your skull. Close your eyes and take a
moment to "grow" the neck, extending
the crown of the head skyward. As you
inhale, open your elbows out to the
sides and back, and extend the neck so
the back of your head moves away from
your shoulders. Cradle your head so you
keep the back of the neck long as you
look up. If you measure where your gaze
arrives, you may notice there is not a large
difference, yet this option probably feels
better on your neck than the previous
one. This feeling of the neck staying
long is what you are aiming for
in backbends like the Cobra and
Locust Poses.

# SHOULDER EXTENSION

These shoulder exercises give more lift with "longer" released arms.

**1.** Stand side-on to the wall, at a distance of about 10 in (25 cm). The more flexible you are, the closer you will get to the wall. Stretch the arm closest to the wall as high up as you can reach, touching your palm to wall. Take several slow breaths, feeling like you are hanging down from the raised hand. Now take it back 45 degrees (pictured) for another ten or so breaths. Finally, take it further behind, to be, if possible, parallel to the floor. Lean your chest forward and breathe. After doing one side, if you relax your arms and then swing them together to join the palms you might find the worked arm "longer" than the other. Repeat on the other side.

**2.** Bring your elbows to the padded edge of a table so they are shoulder-width apart. Step back so your ankles are under your hips and you form a table shape. Bring your palms together and lower the head, if possible, so the neck is in line with the spine. You will feel a stretch in the shoulders. This is table prayer pose. As you hold the position, let the side ribs soften down. After ten breaths here, slowly lower your hands between your shoulder blades so your fingers point toward your tail bone. Move slowly between these two positions a few times. To come up, walk in, lift your head and scoop up.

# SUPTA VIRASANA **Reclining Hero Pose**

The iliopsoas is a deep muscle running from the inner thigh bone to the lumbar vertebrae. When this muscle is tight or contracted, it pulls us into a forward bend. A released iliopsoas muscle is essential for healthy backbending. Begin in Virasana (*see* page 53). Lean back on your elbows, then come up a little so you can lift your pubic bone up as you stretch your tail bone away. Breathe here for a while. Maintaining the tilt of the pelvis, keep your floating ribs from jutting out as you lower your buttocks to the floor. Gaze straight ahead or take the head back and stretch the chin away. If this stretch is too strong on the thighs, practice the lunge outlined in the first part of Anjaneyasana (*see* page 72), and Virabhadrasana I (*see* page 38).

# 21 ANJANEYASANA CRESCENT MOON POSE

The iliopsoas-lengthening lunge part of this pose is a good warm-up for all the other backbends. There are two directions of movement of energy in this pose. The movement from the back of the waist down extends out through the back foot and allows the hips to descend. The upward stretch beginning at the waist radiates energy upward.

**1.** Kneel on a cushioned surface and step your left leg forward. Cup the floor with your fingertips and bring the hips forward to lunge. Ground through the back knee as you allow time and the breath to further open the left groin and lower the hips. Give the muscles time to relax in this pose. When you have connected to the grounding force of gravity and the hips have got the message to drop, lower the chest down slightly, lengthen forward with the breastbone, press the fingertips to the floor, and lift up to increase the bend in the back. Then practice on the other side.

1

**2.** Return to lunge on the first side. When you have followed the same steps, bring your hands to your front knee. Then reach the arms forward and cross the fingers for strength. Lift the upper body up to the sky. Imagine someone is gently pulling you by your wrists up out of your hips. At the same time, release the hips so they sink more to the floor. If the pressure of your back knee against the floor is uncomfortable, press down more through the top of the back foot. If you are comfortable and feel you have a good lifting sensation, proceed to the next step.

## EXPLORE

The thoracic region bends back less easily than the lumbar and cervical regions. Remain aware of where you are working from when practicing backbends. Otherwise you will be at risk of overworking the lower back and neck and underworking the mid and upper back. Extend and arch the whole spine evenly to avoid compressing the spaces between the vertebrae.

2

**3.** Lengthen the spine further, then lift the breastbone up, curve the back backward, and bring the shoulders and arms back. Drop the head back and stretch the chin away. Inhale to come out of the pose and repeat with the right leg forward.

3

# USTRASANA CAMEL POSE

Forming the camel's hump strongly stretches the thighs, opens the groin and lifts the heart. The fifth chakra at the throat is activated in this posture where the head is tilted back and the chin stretched away.

**1.** Kneel with your knees hip-width apart. Place your right hand on your lower back and stretch the other one straight up in the air. Push your hips forward and lift up the breastbone. Use the raised arm to give you a lift as you extend back. Keep the head and neck in line with the upper arm and breathe freely. Repeat on the other side before sitting down on the heels.

1

**2.**  While kneeling, tuck your toes under. This
time, lift up well through the top arm and
bring the other arm down so your fingers
hold the heel. Don't twist the body. Keep both
hips and front ribs facing forward. After five
breaths, repeat on the second side.

**3.**  Now you are warmed up for the full Ustrasana. From kneeling,
take both hands to the small of your back and massage it a little.
The energy moves down from the back of the waist to ground
through the knees. Remember the feeling of lift that the raised
arms gave to the first two exercises. Maintain the lift through the
spine from the back of the waist upward to open the chest. Take
the hands one by one to the heels. Then use them as your anchor
to open the groin and stretch the hips forward, aiming to have
the thigh bones vertical. Continue to lift the breastbone to the
sky as you roll your shoulders back. Finally, take your head back.
When it is time to come up, pressurize your feet on the floor,
inhale and come up. After three repetitions, release the back by
using Balasana or Child Pose (*see* page 21).

2

3

## EXPLORE

You can increase the challenge of this
pose by untucking the toes so that
the tops of the feet are on the floor.
To further deepen the pose, bring the
knees and feet together. Remember
that both the front and back sides of
the body must participate equally in
the backbends. Exhale and soften the
face to release tension.

# SETU BANDHASANA BRIDGE POSE

23

Strengthen your body and expand your heart center in this pose.

1

**1.** Lie on your back with your knees bent up. Have your knees and feet body-width apart. Lift your pelvis slightly so your buttocks just begin to move off the ground. As you take several breaths in this position, lengthen your tail bone toward your feet. Now peel your vertebrae, one by one, off the floor. Tuck the shoulders, under one by one, and move the breastbone toward the chin.

**2.** While the breastbone moves toward your chin, the tailbone moves toward the knees and the knees stretch away from you. Don't let your knees splay apart—keep them only as wide as your hips by squeezing the inner thighs toward each other. Check that excess tension is not building up in the neck. After holding five to ten breaths, come down and rest. Repeat twice more. Then hug the knees into the chest and rock from side to side to release the back.

2

## EXPLORE

If you can straighten your elbows, then interlace the fingers and press the arms down. If your body is ready for more of a challenge, grasp your ankles with your hands. Have patience as you approach each new edge in a pose. Respect the body and wait for it to let you in.

# MATSYASANA FISH POSE

24

Matsyasana is a good pose for releasing the neck after practicing Shoulderstand (*see* page 110), Plough Pose (*see* page 114), and Knee to Ear Pose (*see* page 115).

**1.** Sit on the floor with your legs in front. For this whole sequence you need to press the insides of the feet and thighs together. Lean back on your hands and pressurize the palms to the floor. Lengthen the arms and lift up with the chest. Fully engage your mind in this process. Take your head back and don't forget to breathe. Lift the head and inhale as you come up out of the pose.

1

3

**2.** If you would like to take it a step further, lean back on your elbows so your fingers are by your buttocks. Press down into the elbows and lift the chest into a beautiful arch. With each inhalation, feel the spine move into the core of the body and elongate, setting it up for you to deepen the pose on the exhalation.

**3.** From position 2, slide your elbows apart to lower down on the crown of your head. Stretch your arms overhead, and reach the fingers away actively. To release, bring the arms to your sides, inhale to lift the head slightly, and then slide it away and lie flat.

# EXPLORE

Bring your mental sensitivity to the back of the body; feel how it stretches and the skin thins out.

# URDVA DHANURASANA
## UPWARD-FACING BOW POSE

25

Many people who have difficulty rising up into this pose assume that it is because they lack strength but often it is due to a lack of shoulder flexibility. If your shoulders are tight, then first practice releasing the shoulders with the table prayer pose from the section on alignment (*see* Shoulder Extension 2 on page 71). Prepare for this demanding pose with Crescent Moon Pose (*see* page 72) to open the groin and stretch the thighs.

1

**1.** Lie on your back, with your knees bent up. The action on the back is better when the feet are not turned out so check that your toes are pointing forward. Place your palms near the shoulders, fingers pointing in the direction of the hips. Hold here as you allow the anchoring of the heels to earth to take place. Fully feeling the weight of the heels, slowly peel the back up off the floor and lift the hips. Let the grounding of the body come through the heels, then down into the earth.

## CAUTION

This pose is not advisable in cases of slipped disk, hernia, heart problems and high blood pressure, during menstruation, pregnancy, or in the postnatal period.

2

**2.** Watching the breath, wait for the inner cue to move. Catch it when it comes by lifting your hips as you pressurize the palms and straighten the arms to lift your body into the full position.

**3.** Now you are up, adjust your feet, which may have turned out. Press your inner thighs closer together. As in Bridge Pose (*see* page 76), push the groin up. Let the spine move in toward the front of the body while you consolidate the pose, then expand it in both directions away from the back of the waist. It might help to lengthen toward the tail bone if you lift your heels off the ground for a few breaths.

## EXPLORE

Your yoga practice is not just how you look in a pose. It is how you are when you are not in it, too. This includes going into and coming out of a pose. Never collapse out of a pose, but maintain a steady control. When resting in between repetitions, take your awareness to the back of the body (including the back of the brain) and you will recover more quickly.

# AFTER BACKBENDING

26

Always practice a couple of twists and forward bends after a session on backbending.

## ROCKING

Your back will enjoy this massage. Lying down, hug your knees into your chest and rock slowly from side to side. Then press your knees away, resisting with your arms. More of your lower back will come into contact with the floor as you rock.

## BHARADVAJASANA  Sage Twist I

Spiraling outward and upward releases tension from the whole torso.

## PASSIVE OPENING OUT TWIST

Stretching out like a starfish expands the heart.

## BALASANA Child Pose

This relaxing pose cultivates the sense of release and surrender.

## YOGAMUDRASANA Sealing Pose

This pose quietens the mind and is very comfortable.

## PASSIVE RECLINING TWIST

Let the softness inherent in this pose release the back.

## PASCHIMOTTANASANA

Stretch out the back and hamstrings in this pose.

# TWISTS

From where you're sitting, twist around to one side for ten breaths. Wind yourself up tight. Coil around with every cell in your torso. Now uncoil. Feel different? A twist is a great opportunity to turn and see things from a different angle.

When you feel wound up by life, temporarily increase the winding with a twist. Spiral up to the sky, then feel the tension dissipate as you undo and consciously unwind out of the twist.

The vertebrae are held in place by many small muscles and ligaments that need to be exercised to stay in top shape. Should they weaken, or should the distribution of strength through the back be uneven, the spine can be pulled out of alignment. A decrease of innervation can cause all sorts of problems in other areas and body systems.

An often-used analogy is that of the dish sponge. When the sponge is full of soapy water, it can be squeezed out, ready to fill with clean water. That's what twists do to the abdominal organs. They temporarily increase the pressure on them so that the deoxygenated blood is squeezed out. Then the organs receive fresh oxygen and nutrient-rich blood.

Our wellbeing depends on a happy spine. Twists prevent stiffness of the spine and counteract any decrease in mobility that makes one look and feel old. Wringing out the body releases lots of built-up tension. Twists can reduce headaches and stiffness in the neck and shoulders. Depending on the cause, they can work miracles in relieving backache, as they stretch and strengthen the tiny muscles that link each vertebra to its neighbor. They help the spine maintain a healthy alignment. Twists nourish the disks between the vertebrae. As the intervertebral disks have no direct blood supply from adulthood on, the bending forward, backward, and twisting of yoga postures brings them the nutrients they need to keep healthy. When practicing twists, take some time to lengthen the torso first to be sure you are elongating, not compressing the spine.

Twists increase vitality, energy, and boost the flow of prana around the body. By placing pressure on the organs of digestion, then releasing it, twists feed the digestive fire. Through their massaging effect on the organs, they eliminate sluggishness and ward off constipation.

Don't practice twists intensively if you have a hernia or have had recent surgery; consult an experienced teacher first. Proceed with extreme caution if you have disk problems, as the twists will need to be implemented gradually, allowing for any delayed feedback from your body. Women benefit from practicing twists between periods to relieve menstrual cramps. During menstruation, use gentle twists. In pregnancy, practice simple twists in an open way (for example, without compressing the abdomen against the thigh) and flow in and out of them a few times without holding for long.

*Above and opposite:* A twist offers a mental break and a time to view things from a fresh perspective.

# BHARADVAJASANA I

27

## SAGE TWIST I

Spiraling outward and upward releases tension from the whole torso.

**1.** From Dandasana (*see* page 52), bring your legs around to the left and tuck the right foot under the left ankle. Have both knees facing forward. Hold your right knee with your left hand. Bring your right hand to the floor behind you. Sink the sitting bones toward the floor, and take as many breaths as you need to extend up from your base. If this starting position is not at all comfortable for you, place a small support like a cushion or folded blanket under one buttock to level yourself off.

1

2

**2.** When you have lengthened well, revolving from the hips, spiral into the fuller twist, moving with the support of your abdominal organs. If possible, slide your left hand under the knee, wrist facing out. Catch hold of your left arm with your right hand and look back over your shoulder. More advanced practitioners can anchor down well through the left sitting bone, allowing the shortened left side of the waist to elongate as the right naturally does. After five to ten breaths, sit on your heels to rest and feel the effects, before repeating on side two.

## EXPLORE

Bring your head into the pose just as you would normally. Measure with your eyes how far around you go. Now turn just your neck and head back to the front. This time, close your eyes and, with awareness, bring your neck and head back around into the twist. Go only as far as feels healthily comfortable for your neck. Open your eyes and note how far you reached.

# JATHARA PARIVARTANASANA

## REVOLVED ABDOMEN POSE

28

Weak abdominal muscles often contribute to chronic back pain. This exercise, practiced daily, will quickly strengthen the muscles. The passive reclining twist is less strengthening, but wonderful for easing pain caused by tight back muscles pulling on the vertebrae and causing nerve irritation and pain.

**Passive Reclining Twist**

**1.** Lie on your back with your knees bent up close to the chest. Take your arms out to the sides. Keep your knees in close to the body and slowly drop both your knees over to the right side, aiming them toward your elbow. Relax both knees and feet down to the floor. If your knees or feet don't arrive there, rest them on a folded blanket. Turn your head to the left side. There is nothing more to do in this pose. Bring your attention to actively undoing the parts of the body that are holding on to tension. Check the buttocks, back, shoulders, and face. Stay in this pose for one to two minutes. To come up, turn your head back to center first, lift the top leg in the air, then the other leg, then proceed to side two.

1

## EXPLORE

You can move the emphasis of the passive twist up and down the back depending on where you place your knees. If your thighs are more at right angles with the torso, the emphasis of the twist is further down the back. If your knees start close to your chest and land close to your elbow, the twist moves up the back.

**2.** Build toward the full pose with an intermediate exercise. Lie on your back with your arms out to the sides, hands at shoulder level. Bring both legs up in the air. Lift the hips and "bunny hop" the buttocks to the left. While extending out through both heels, hold the left leg steady and exhale your right leg out to the side, aiming your toes toward the fingertips. On your next exhalation, slowly lower your left leg to join the right. Inhale your left leg back to vertical and on your next inhalation, raise the right leg. Complete five repetitions on each side, following the flow of the breath. Bend your knees if necessary.

2

**3.** If your legs can come to at least a 90-degree angle, then you are ready for the full pose with straight legs. If, when you raise your legs in the air, they don't come at least to vertical, keep your knees bent as you follow these instructions. "Bunny hop" your buttocks 6 in (15 cm) to the left, so that your toes angle off toward the right hand. Exhale to lower both legs to the right at the same time. If you can, catch hold of the feet. Your top heel will usually sit behind the other. To increase the twist, reach the top heel away as you "revolve" your abdominal muscles in the opposite direction. Anchor as much of the left side of your trunk and left shoulder to the floor as you can. Turn your head to gaze at your left hand. Do an even number of repetitions on each side, exhaling down and inhaling up. For the final repetition, stay in this twist for five breaths before inhaling up.

3

# 29

# PASSIVE OPENING OUT TWIST

Stretching out like a starfish expands the heart.
Open yourself to a childlike feeling of happiness.

**1**. Lie on your front with your arms and legs apart like a star. Your
right hand and both your feet will stay attached to the floor, and
your left arm will move.

## EXPLORE

In this position, one lung is more open than the other. Explore
the expansion of the side ribs with each inhalation as the air is
drawn more into that side of the chest and it is exercised fully.

2

**2.** As you bring your arm up and over, let your left hip come up. Allow your knees to bend gently and roll over more onto the sides of your feet. Turn the head to look behind you. Your left arm and shoulder might stay floating in the air. Either use gravity, patience, and the breath to ease them down or, if you like, rest them on a folded blanket. In time, gravity will assist the easing down process. If your left shoulder can touch the floor, stretch the other shoulder away to increase the distance between them.

3

**3.** Rest in this position for one to two minutes, tuning into the purity of the heart center. Before you move on to do the same on the other side, rest like the starfish, or in Makrasana (see page 123) to observe what has been mobilized on the physical, mental, and/or emotional levels.

# MARICHYASANA III SAGE TWIST III

30

This twist develops shoulder flexibility, tones the abdominal organs, and stimulates sluggish intestinal function. This pose is named after Marichi, who, like Bharadvaja, was a man of great wisdom.

**1.** Sit in Dandasana (*see* page 52). Bend the left knee up so that your heel comes close to your buttock. Before planting the seed of "twisting" in the mind, allow yourself to grow taller. Lean back on your left hand and reach your right hand up to the sky. Take as many breaths as necessary to "grow" both sides of the torso.

## EXPLORE

The breath tends to shorten and feel more labored in this twist. Consciously smooth and round out the breath.

1

**2.** This next part is crucial. You need to lean forward and wedge your right elbow to the left outer knee without losing the length you have just gained. Do this movement consciously, over one or more exhalations, taking care not to shorten the left side of the torso. Twist in sections from the base up. Twist on the exhale until you reach the chest, and then twist on the inhale. Feel yourself twisting from the inside out; from the inner organs to the outer casing of your body. Hold for five to ten breaths, then untwist, re-center, and repeat on the other side.

2

**3.** For the full posture, straighten your left arm forward. Reach well forward as if you were taking your armpit beyond the left outer knee. From the shoulder, rotate the whole arm so that the thumb turns down, and wrap your arm around the left knee. Clasp the right wrist behind your back, or work your hands toward each other using a soft belt. As you breathe deeply in this pose, the pressure of your thigh against your abdomen gives the organs a healthy massage.

3

# BALANCES

Our lives feel better when they are well balanced. We are healthiest when
we find the appropriate balance in the food we eat. We feel best when we
find the right levels of activity and sleep. Intellectual balance means we
are able to see both sides of the coin, and be less judgemental.

Emotionally, we seek to lessen extremes of emotions, decrease
mood swings, and be more even-tempered. Spiritual balance lets
us keep higher ideals in mind as our actions create our lives, yet
still allows us to keep our feet on the ground. A spiritual belief
balances and gives meaning to our physical existence. Being
out of balance is a huge source of stress and tends to create
problems. Your yoga practice is a metaphor for your life. Finding
your balance in a pose is practice at finding your balance in your
life. Yoga, as a re-harmonizer, helps you move closer to your own
perfect balance.

Balance poses convey self-sufficiency. Standing on your own
two feet does more than just develop the small muscles of the
ankles. Balancing poses allow us to explore our connection with
our base. In India, the lotus flower is a powerful symbol. The
white flower is a symbol of purity. It floats on top of
its stem, a long taproot that is anchored in deep,
dark waters. Like the lotus flower, we sink our
roots into the earth, and soar skyward. Balance
poses allow you to connect to your roots and
explore whether they feel strong, independent,
and able to support your growth.

Some poses look simple but actually present a real
challenge. All balance poses require that the mind and body work
together. The focused mind collaborates with the grounded body.
Aside from developing concentration and stamina, the poses
develop patience. Don't be in a hurry. Decide for how many
breaths you will stay in the pose, then stay. If you come out early,
keep a quiet mind and bring yourself back into it again.

Arm balances develop endurance. They work the shoulder
girdle, which helps balance out office-bound people. By building
strength in the upper body, they redistribute tension in a healthy
way, which helps decrease neck tension. Developing the arms
enables us to reach out in life, either to take what we need or to
give what we can.

Balance poses teach us about relaxing in all the other
postures. Try balancing when holding your body tight. It will feel
very different from when you proceed in a soft, easy manner that
brings a lightness into your pose. Use the skeleton rather than
tensed muscles to support you. As your mind stays calm and
centered and develops the ability to lead the body, your
co-ordination will grow. Developing physical poise will foster
mental harmony.

*Above and opposite:* Being out of balance creates stress. Yoga
practice helps you move closer to a balanced way of living.

# 31 UTTHITA HASTA PADANGUSTHASANA

## HAND TO FOOT POSE

When a balance pose is a challenge to flexibility, it is amazing how we are forced to focus to stay up. This is good practice.

**1.** Stand in Tadasana (*see* page 36) and ground yourself through your heels. Quieten the mind so that you can fully focus on what you are doing right here and now: this balance. Gaze at a fixed point at eye level. Bend the right knee slightly and pause to let your left leg better connect with the earth. Lift up your right leg and hold the knee with your right hand. With your left hand to your hip, lift the sternum so your posture stays erect. Lengthen the right side waist by moving the right hip down level with the left. Pressing the knee closer to the torso, hold for seven even breaths.

**2.** Now open the leg out to the right. Roving eyes will distract you by taking your awareness elsewhere. Turn your head to gaze left and keep your eyes steady. If you are holding your knee, lift it toward your armpit. If you are holding your toe (*see* alternative opposite), lift it as high as you can. Keep the supporting leg straight. Breathe here for seven rounds. Then, still balancing, bring the leg back to the front. Release the leg and straighten it in midair. Lower the leg slowly and practice the other side.

1

2

1

2

## ALTERNATIVE

If your hamstrings are flexible, loop your big toe with the thumb and finger, and straighten the leg out in front (1). Now keep both sides of the torso an even length by rolling the outer right hip down with an external rotation of the thigh bone (2).

## CAUTION

During pregnancy, practice standing balances near a wall so there is no risk of falling.

## EXPLORE

To build hamstring flexibility, stand in front of a table and place your heel on it. Level the hips by lowering the raised leg side.

# GARUDASANA EAGLE POSE

3 2

This pose develops concentration and co-ordination and is wonderful for tight shoulders.

## EXPLORE

Feel free to practice the upper and lower body movements independently, before uniting them in Garudasana.

**1.** From Tadasana (*see* page 36), become aware of the skin on the soles of the feet widening out against the floor. Move your attention to the pressure of the right foot against the floor. Quietly let the skin of the foot melt down into it. Bend the left knee and lift up the right leg.

**2.** Use momentum to wrap the right leg around the left leg. If you have difficulty with this, bend the supporting leg more. If possible, keep the top knee facing forward, not turned outward. To wrap the arms, hug yourself with your left arm on top of the right. Keeping the cross at the elbows, bring the backs of the hands toward each other, then cross wrist and forearm to bring the palms together.

**3.** Lift the elbows up so they rise off the chest and free breath is not impeded. To stretch into the shoulders more, ease your forearms forward so your thumbs move away from your nose. Let your eagle fold forward, as if looking down on the world from a great height. When you breathe deeply, you will feel the skin between the shoulder blades stretch on each inhalation. Hold the pose for ten breaths, before unwrapping, re-grounding and repeating on the opposite side.

1

2

# VIRABHADRASANA III WARRIOR III

**33**

Let your warrior-like determination give you a mental surge to charge the body with energy.

1

**1.** Assume the pose for Virabhadrasana I with your right foot forward (*see* page 38).

**2.** Inhale deeply and, on the exhalation, fold your torso over your front leg, lowering your ribs toward your thigh. On a strong inhalation, straighten the right leg and lift the back leg up to parallel with the floor. Gaze straight ahead. Keeping your right leg straight, lower your left hip down so it is even with the right. Turn your left toes from the side down toward the floor and extend back through the heel. (You can even place your hands on the back of a chair to practice the alignment.) Visualize a line of energy running along the body. From the back of the waist it extends forward, reaching out toward the fingertips. From your center, it extends backward through the back heel, so everything from heel to fingertips unkinks and elongates. Hold for five breaths before coming gracefully back to Virabhadrasana I.

2

## EXPLORE

Before coming into a pose, close your eyes and visualize yourself clearly in a strong, stable, steady pose.

# BHUJAPIDASANA

## 34

## ARM PRESSURE BALANCE

Despite appearances, this pose doesn't require more upper body strength than you already have. Technique is all-important. With attention to proper positioning and a positive mental attitude, you will be well on your way to balancing.

### EXPLORE

Should your wrists need strengthening, practice Adho Mukha Svanasana (see page 104). To counterstretch the arms after Bhujapidasana, Bakasana, or Adho Mukha Svanasana, kneel and place the backs of the hands on the floor, fingers facing toward your knees. Move the hips back about 2 in (5 cm). Feel the welcome release along the wrists and forearms as you lean back.

**1.** Stand with the feet hip-width apart. As you fold forward, bend the knees but keep your hips high in the air. Take the right arm through the legs and around the right leg. A common error is not to take the whole arm—up to the shoulder—through the legs. It is important that the back of the thigh contacts as high up the upper arm as possible so use your other hand to stabilize you if necessary. Place the right palm flat on the floor just next to the right foot with fingers facing forward. Now take the left arm through to bring that palm flat to the floor. You'll need to keep the hips high so you don't squash your upper arm and get stuck halfway in, unable to proceed.

**2.** Bending your elbows well, lean forward. Inch your feet together and forward. Lift up through the abdominal region and raise your head to gaze forward. Shift your weight to transfer more weight to the palms as you lift your feet up in the air to cross the ankles. Straighten the arms and hold for five to ten breaths. After resting, repeat with the feet crossed the opposite way.

1

2

# BAKASANA CRANE POSE

This pose, resembling a bird, strengthens the upper body and abdomen.

1

2

**1.** Squat with your feet together. Place your hands on the floor as wide as your shoulders, middle fingers facing forward. Bend your knees to rest them high up the upper arms, wrapping your inner knees around the upper arms. Bring the feet together and come onto your tiptoes.

**2.** Lean forward to allow the transfer of weight from toes to palms. Gaze forward along the floor. Lift the abdominal muscles and use yogic energy locks to give your body lift and lightness. One at a time, or together, raise the feet toward the buttocks. Keep your abdominal muscles contracted to help draw the legs into the body. Straighten your arms. Take five breaths before coming down with control.

## EXPLORE

As you commit to a pose, you agree to go on a journey and appreciate what it has to offer you. When practicing balancing poses, decide first for how many breaths you will stay and keep to it.

# INVERSIONS

Holding a position with a whole new relationship to gravity demands a certain steadiness of posture and mind. Inversions develop confidence and help quiet the brain in times of stress.

Inversions are key poses for regaining hormonal balance, as better blood circulation tones the endocrine glands. In particular, Headstand tones the pituitary and pineal glands in the brain, both of which have wide-ranging effects in the body. Shoulderstand and Plough Pose bring blood to the thyroid and parathyroid glands by the throat.

The lymphatic system, involved in immune support and clearing toxins from the tissues, reaps the benefits from anti-gravity positions. The lymphatic vessels don't have any valves or muscles to help pump their fluid through. The passive flow instead relies on changes in position and massaging movements from the muscles surrounding them. Going upside down helps drain toxins from the extremities down toward their destination: the lymph nodes. The lymphatic fluid drains in the direction of the heart and, by assisting this process, inverted poses relieve strain or swelling in the legs and clear the path for improved blood circulation.

Inversions are even considered aerobic, as the heart must pump harder to pump out the more rapidly filling ventricles. The functioning of the organs is stimulated by the change in position and circulation, and intestinal laziness is lessened by the alteration in internal pressure.

When you feel stuck, or in need of inspiration, it helps to see the world from another angle. Releasing the pressure of our normal reality—gravity—can lighten the mind, too. An upside-down position is an opportunity to consider things from a different point of view. Apart from being mentally revitalizing and rejuvenating, inversions have the same physical action. By cleansing and nourishing the tissues, many people swear by their effects at maintaining youthfulness. As a sort of holistic beauty treatment, they might be the closest you can get to turning back the clock.

If you suffer high blood pressure, a neck problem, eye, ear or sinus problems, heart problems, hiatus hernia, or dizzy spells, seek advice from a medical practitioner or experienced yoga teacher before beginning inversions. During pregnancy, work with an experienced teacher. Inversions are not advisable during menstruation, as they tend to slow down the flow of blood. Don't practice inverted poses if you have a headache at the time. As inversions are considered calming to the mind and cooling to the system, they are generally used toward the end of your asana practice, and when your body has been warmed by the other poses.

*Above and opposite: Inverted poses clear the head and help concentration. The brain receives an increased blood supply, combating tiredness and lethargy.*

# ADHO MUKHA SVANASANA

## DOWNWARD-FACING DOG

This is an excellent pose for stretching and strengthening the whole body. This forward-folding mild inversion is useful to link standing poses. Although it may not feel very restful at first, it can become so when you develop strength and flexibility.

If, instead of being relatively straight, your back rounds in the full Downward-Facing Dog, practice Puppy Dog. As a gentler way to open the shoulders, you can hold and breathe in this pose longer. If wrist problems prevent you doing the full pose at this time, begin with this easier version.

**1.** Begin on all fours with your hands placed about 6 in (15 cm) in front of the shoulders. Check that the middle finger is pointing straight ahead, and spread the fingers wide.

**2.** Have your knees and feet body-width apart. Tuck the toes under and lift up to an inverted V-position. On tiptoes, bend both knees deeply, so your ribs come toward the thighs, or even touch. You will feel an increase in the stretch through the shoulders and an opening in the chest. At the same time, lift the sitting bones as the buttocks stay high and tilt the pelvis forward. The inward curve in the lower back will deepen as your navel moves closer to your thighs. (This pose is also a forward bend, so refresh your body's memory about folding from the hips: *see* page 37.) You will feel the muscles along the spine working strongly and get a lifting sense of elongation along the spine.

**3.** Keeping the hips at the same height, slowly straighten the legs. If the hips stay at, or nearly at, the same height, everything in between will need to lengthen. Practice this several times, with full awareness, so you don't lose the feeling of height or the inward curve in the lower back. To complete, swivel your feet so the outside edges of your feet are parallel—the inner heels will be further away from each other than the big toes. Stretch your heels toward the ground (until you develop a lot of flexibility along the backs of the legs, they will remain in the air). Distribute the pressure equally through the whole palm and fingers. Widen the space between the earlobes and upper arms by turning the outer edges of the armpits in toward each other. Hold for 10 to 15 breaths. Rest in Child Pose (*see* page 21) afterward. Soften the arms from the shoulders all the way to the wrists. To release the wrists, follow the instructions on page 100.

3

# ALTERNATIVE **Puppy Dog**

This gentler version of Downward-Facing Dog gives the shoulders a good stretch. Kneel on the floor. Place your hands far forward and lower your forehead to the floor. Have your knees under your hips so your buttocks are high in the air, not near the heels. From the back of the waist, extend back strongly through the tail bone. At the same time direct your energy from the waist forward through the arms.

# ALTERNATIVE **Raised Leg Variation**

To make this pose into a stronger inversion, start with your feet together. Turn the right toes out and lift the right leg high up in the air. Keep both shoulders level. Let your right hip rise up and extend back through both heels. After five to ten breaths, lower the leg and stretch through both legs (or rest in Child Pose—*see* page 21) before practicing the other side.

# SIRSASANA HEADSTAND

37

Your head weighs about 9 lb (4 kg), your body considerably more. Your neck can hold the weight of your head only when you are properly prepared. It is essential to understand the lifting through the shoulders and pay due attention to alignment. This is not a beginner's pose and I strongly recommend you ask an experienced teacher to observe your alignment. If Headstand is not yet for you, the Hare Pose (*see* page 109) is a possible alternative.

Headstand is a yogic icon, often the first pose people think of when they first hear of yoga. Ironically, you must get your head out of the way in Headstand. If you want to do this classic pose just because your ego wants to do "real yoga," it doesn't necessarily mean your body is ready to follow. Practice Headstand well into your practice when your body is warm. Before going up, visualize yourself in the posture. Form a clear picture of yourself in a steady, stable pose.

**1.** Always practice Headstand on a cushioned surface like a folded blanket. Place your blanket in front of a wall, or in the corner of two walls. Kneel in front of your blanket. To measure out the correct elbow-width, place your forearms on the blanket and cup each elbow in the opposite hand. Your elbows should be not wider than your shoulders. Then form your triangle of support by interlacing your fingers together. Your knuckles should be 2 in (5 cm) from the wall.

1

**2.** When performing a safe Headstand, it is crucial to lift well from elbows to shoulders. Tuck your toes under and straighten your knees so you are in an inverted V-shape. Practice your lift by pressing down through the elbows and moving the shoulders up toward the hips. This movement should increase the distance between the shoulders and earlobes as well as lifting the head away from the floor. If you find you can't lift your head away from the floor, you are not ready for Headstand yet. You need to develop your shoulder flexibility and/or strength before attempting to go up into Headstand. For shoulder flexibility, practice the shoulder exercises on page 71, as well as Gomukhasana (*see* page 64), and Garudasana (*see* page 98). To develop arm strength, practice Downward-Facing Dog (*see* page 104).

**3.** Take your knees back to the floor and position your head on the floor to be cupped by your interlaced fingers. For the correct alignment in the neck, it is the crown of the head that should be in contact with the floor. Once again raise the knees off the floor and practice moderating the pressure on the head. Ground down through the elbows, distribute weight into the edges of the hands against the floor, lift the shoulders up toward the hips. If you are not able to minimize the pressure on the crown of the head with these actions, then don't move on to the next step. Develop this skill with more preparatory work before you come up into Headstand.

2

4

**4.** If you have passed these checks, then walk your feet in as much as possible. There will come a point where the feet naturally want to lift. Lift them with knees bent so your heels come near your buttocks. Don't raise the legs all the way up straight away. Follow these steps to help your alignment stay true. Lift up from your elbows through your shoulders to your hips once more.

**5.** If you are not using a wall and feel balanced, keep your knees bent and raise the thighs so the knees point upward. Your heels will still be near your buttocks. Then straighten your legs up. If you are by a wall, straighten your legs and lift upward through the balls of the feet.

5

## CAUTION

Headstand, Shoulderstand, Halasana, and Karnapidasana should not be practiced during menstruation or with some ear or eye problems, like detached retina or glaucoma. For heart problems, high blood pressure, previous neck injuries, or pregnancy, seek the advice of an experienced teacher.

6

**6.** Check that your floating ribs are not jutting out—lengthen the back of the waist to bring them in. Should your shoulders be collapsing and causing the head to bear more than a little pressure, come down immediately. Energize the back of the body, too. In the beginning hold for five breaths. Over many months, slowly build your holding time to up to five minutes. Come down by reversing the steps you took to go up. Always rest in Child Pose afterward and follow on with Shoulderstand.

## ALTERNATIVE Hare Pose

If Headstand if not yet for you, this is a possible alternative. Begin in Child Pose (*see* page 21). Hold the sides of your feet with your hands. Lifting the buttocks high, inhale and roll over your head onto the crown. On the exhalation, release back to Child Pose. Repeat five times.

# SARVANGASANA SHOULDERSTAND

38

This hormonal balancing and deeply calming pose is well worth practicing daily.

**1.** To keep your neck relaxed in this pose, fold two or three blankets to the size that will support your base. Place the folded edges neatly, one on top of the other. Lie over them with your head on the lower level, and the tops of your shoulders on your blankets, 2 in (5 cm) from the edge.

**2.** With control, bring your legs and hips in the air and then support your back. If your stomach muscles are not yet strong enough to bring you up, or if you can't yet come up in a well-controlled way that feels safe, use the wall method. Once you are up, bend your knees toward your head. Take several breaths to settle your shoulders into the pose. Let yourself come more onto the tips of the well-grounded shoulders and walk the hands down your back. Finally, stretch your legs up into the air. In the beginning, your legs may be angled to be quite bent overhead, not straight up in the air. Bring your elbows closer together. You may get a better grip holding your palms against the skin on your back rather than your clothes. In time, work on lessening the crease where the thighs join the torso. Visualize a line of energy from the inner thigh to the inner heel.

1

2

**3.** Never turn the head from side to side in this pose. Shoulderstand is not called neckstand for good reason! Although it might look like the neck is taking a lot of weight, the neck muscles need to stay relatively soft. If possible, ask a friend to touch the muscles on either side of your neck to check they are not strained tight. Likewise, redness or strain in the face means it's time to come down and rest. Build your time in the pose from one to up to ten minutes.

**4.** After Shoulderstand, you can practice Halasana or Karnapidasana (pages 114 and 115 respectively). To come down, use the abdominal muscles to lower yourself down in a slow, controlled way. Slide off the blankets and lie flat. Release your neck by turning your head from side to side. The lower back and abdominal organs will probably communicate some different sensations to you, so practice with a twist and a forward bend afterward. A nice sequence starts with Matsyasana (*see* page 78) to release the neck. Then hug your knees to your chest and rock slowly from side to side. Follow with Passive Reclining Twist (*see* page 88), which works wonderfully after Shoulderstand. Finally practice Paschimottanasana (*see* page 56).

# SHOULDERSTAND AGAINST THE WALL

This controlled, step-by-step way of lifting into Shoulderstand in stages is a good way to start feeling comfortable with Shoulderstand.

**1.** Place your folded blankets a little away from the wall—as your head needs to be off the blankets but your shoulders supported by them, you may have to experiment to find the correct width for the length of your body. If you have a non-slip yoga mat, place it on top of the blankets. Sit side on and up close to the wall. Using your arms for support, slowly bring your legs up and your trunk around and down, to lie over the blankets.

1

**2.** If you have found the right position with your blankets, your head will be on the floor, your shoulders 2 in (5 cm) from the edge of the blankets and your buttocks near the wall. Lift your head and check that your body is symmetrical, perpendicular to the wall.

2

**3.** Now you are ready to come up! With knees bent, press your feet into the wall and lift your hips. Hold your back and straighten yourself up by moving your hips more in line over your shoulders. If you like, you can straighten each leg in turn bringing one foot up the wall. Once you have both legs straight against the wall, take one leg, then the other, overhead and away from the wall. Come down by reversing the steps you took to go up.

## EXPLORE

A few variations keep the mind alert in Shoulderstand. Practice lowering one foot to the floor while keeping the leg extending strongly upward. Alternatively, bring the soles of the feet together and open the knees out in a kind of upside-down Cobbler's Pose. Follow that by opening your legs into a wide V-shape.

3

# HALASANA PLOUGH POSE

If you are comfortable in Shoulderstand, follow on with this soothing pose. It has similar effects and contraindications to Shoulderstand.

**1.** From Shoulderstand lower your legs overhead. You need to be careful not to overstretch the neck as you bring your toes to touch the floor. If you are not able to bring your toes to the floor, then rest them on a higher surface, such as a chair placed a couple of feet behind the head. (If your toes are not supported, then continue to support your back with your hands.)

**2.** Once your toes are resting on a surface, stretch your arms along the floor. This will help you roll more onto the tips of your shoulders and deeper into this upside-down forward bend. Interlace your fingers and deepen the pose by stretching your arms and legs in opposite directions. Build up to holding this pose for five minutes. Make Plough Pose more restful by supporting the thighs with a chair if you wish.

**3.** Roll out of the pose with control, using your abdominal muscles to lower both legs until you are lying flat. See Shoulderstand for complementary asanas to follow on with.

# KARNAPIDASANA KNEE TO EAR POSE

Withdraw into a foetal position after practicing Shoulderstand and Plough Pose.

If you feel comfortable in Halasana, practice this deep forward stretch by cushioning yourself with a couple of folded blankets and bending your knees beside your head. If your knees and tops of the feet don't come to the floor, place your legs on raised supports or tuck your toes under if necessary.

To deepen the pose, straighten both arms along the floor and interlace your fingers. If your knees touch the floor, fold your arms over the backs of your knees. Hold this pose for 10 to 20 breaths before coming back to Halasana.

# Surya Namaskar
## Sun Salutation

**41**

1

2

The Sun Salutation is a group of dynamic yoga postures that flow together to warm the body and work the heart. While you link movement and breath, you stretch and strengthen the muscles, developing stamina, co-ordination and confidence. There are many possible variations of Surya Namaskar to suit all ages and abilities, so ask your teacher for help if necessary.

The sun is a symbol of the inner light that is in all of us. The bowing is an exercise of deep respect for this shining light, the folding and unfolding movements a tribute to creation. As you develop a graceful flow of one movement per breath, it becomes a moving meditation. Start your practice with three rounds and build to six, offering each one up like a prayer. Then sit quietly and listen as your body tells you what it would like to practice next.

**1.** Mountain Pose with palms together, ground through the feet and feel the connection with the earth through the soles of the feet.

**2.** Inhale your arms skyward. As the front of your torso lengthens, keep the back side of the torso long as well.

**3.** Intense Forward Stretch. Exhale and fold forward to touch the earth.

**4.** With fingertips touching the floor (bend your knees if necessary), lunge. Inhale and step your left leg back. Lift your chest away from your thighs.

4

3

5

**5.** Exhale and step your feet back to Plank Pose, forming a straight line from heels to shoulders.

6

**6** Still exhaling, bring your shoulders forward of your wrists, so your elbows form a right angle as you lower your body to 2 in (5 cm) off the floor.

7

8

9

## EXPLORE

Give yourself time to feel your way into the poses by holding each one for several slow breaths. Practice Ujjayi breathing (*see* page 131) during the Sun Salutation.

**7.** Cobra: Lower your body to the floor, then inhale as you press your hands to the floor to curve the chest up in Cobra Pose.

**8.** Downward-Facing Dog: Exhale while you tuck your toes under and lift the hips high. Hold for three breaths.

**9.** Inhale and step the right leg between your hands.

**10.** Intense Forward Stretch. Exhale as you step your left leg forward, then fold over your legs. If your legs are straight, press your hands more to the floor.

**11.** Switch on your thigh muscles and those of the lower abdomen as you inhale skyward. Lift everything from the hips up, except the shoulders.

**12.** Exhale and bring the arms down to Mountain Pose, ready to repeat on the left side.

# RESTORATIVE YOGA

Restorative poses open the body, yet allow the nervous system to rest. Though you can still stretch deeply, the support helps you feel safe and comfortable yielding to the pose, and you can stay in it for longer. It enables you to recharge by expending minimal energy.

As such, these poses are wonderful should you need to build energy stores during a chronic illness or to tap into your inner reserves and rejuvenate whenever you feel depleted.

Incorporate restorative poses into your regular practice routine, either by practicing them a few days each month (they are ideal during menstruation), or by bringing one or two poses into each more active practice session.

To find props around your house, think creatively and use couch cushions, cushions, blankets, chairs, soft belts, and bathrobe ties. An eyebag gives the system a break from sensory overload.

# SUPTA KONASANA

## SUPPORTED ANGLE POSE

This restorative pose creates space in the pelvis, eases menstrual dysfunction for women and supports the digestive system. It is worth folding a pile of blankets to luxuriate in complete comfort in this pose.

Use a bolster or fold up several blankets so they are longer than your torso. Sit at one end of your support and bring the soles of your feet together, heels toward your groin. Lie back over the bolster and have an extra cushion under your head so it is higher than the heart. Let your knees fall out to the sides and use pillows or folded blankets of equal heights to support your thighs. Find the right balance between opening the hips and staying comfortable—if the stretch becomes too intense it will be hard to rest. Cover your body for warmth if necessary. Lay your arms out to the sides, palms facing up. If your elbows don't naturally reach the floor, then fold towels or blankets to support the forearms. Close or cover your eyes and rest for five to ten minutes. When you come up, stretch forward in Child Pose, or a variation of it with your big toes together, knees apart, and arms stretched forward.

# FORWARD BEND WITH A CHAIR

43

The same principle can be used for many forward bends: Trianga Mukhaikapada Paschimottanasana, Janu Sirsasana, Ardha Baddha Padma Paschimottanasana, Paschimottanasana, and Baddha Konasana.

Sit on the edge of a folded blanket with your legs wide apart. Place a second blanket over the seat of a chair. Bring the chair far enough away so that when you fold forward your forehead, will rest on it. To keep the chest open, bring the arms up to hold the chair base or back—experiment to find the most comfortable position. If you feel too much stretch, use cushions to raise the level of your forehead. After some time in the pose, your body will release and you'll find you can slide the chair further away to deepen the stretch. If you are very flexible, then you can rest your forehead on just a bolster or cushions. The gentle pressure on the forehead rests the frontal lobe of the brain, helping to quieten the mind and soothe the soul. Next, in this resting variation of Upavista Konasana, you can do two twists, too. Turn your torso to face over one leg, position the chair over it and fold forward to rest the forehead. Hold each forward bend for one to two minutes.

# VIPARITA KARANI

## RESTORATIVE INVERSION

**44**

Viparita Karani is used to seal life energy in your body. Enjoy the benefits of an inversion without the effort of holding yourself in place. To relieve swelling in the legs after a hard day, or to ease the pain of varicose veins, practice for ten minutes every day. During menstruation, forgo the blankets and simply lie on the floor with the legs up the wall.

Take a bolster or fold several blankets and place them by a wall. To come into the position, sit on your prop and lie yourself down on your side so your buttocks stay high and near the wall. Roll onto your back and take your legs up the wall. Check your position. Your abdomen needs to be parallel to the floor and your ribcage will curve downward. You may need to experiment a bit to get the right height and width in your blankets. If either is wrong, it will feel like you might slide off and you won't be able to relax properly. When the position feels perfect, look along your body to check that your trunk is perpendicular to the wall. If you like, tie a soft belt around the mid-thighs so your legs don't have to work to hold their position. You can cover your eyes with an eyebag. Choose a comfortable arm position— either slightly away from your sides with your palms facing up, or with the arms overhead and elbows softly bent.
Rest and breathe.

# MAKRASANA CROCODILE POSE

45

This resting position has a gentle backbend so it is useful for resting without breaking the flow in between stronger backbends. Experiment to find the angle of the upper arms that will give you the perfect feeling of the right amount of backbend and the right angle for the resting neck and head.

Lie face down with your feet wide apart and toes turned out. Cup each elbow in the opposite hand and slide the forearms away so they are a short distance in front of your shoulders. Lower your head to rest your forehead on your forearms. Each time you inhale, your abdomen will expand down into the earth. Become attuned to the soothing sensation of this massage. This position is also useful to feel the expansion and consolidation along the back of the torso with each breath.

## EXPLORE

A forward-bending restorative pose, which also creates a belly massage and permits the expansion of the back ribs, is Child Pose (see page 21).

## NOTE

Savasana relaxation (see page 22), Discovering the Breath (see page 132), and letting yourself hang down in the Roll Downs (see page 32) are also restorative practices.

# YOGA ON A CHAIR

These make great office exercises and they are useful for the elderly or infirm. If you are at work, shut the door and take your phone off the hook to give yourself the best chance for full mental relaxation.

## BACKBEND

Different chairs will give you stretches of various intensities at different points along the spine, so experiment to find the best one for you. The chair back should be below or level with the lower part of your shoulder blades. If your chair is high-backed, sit on telephone directories to raise your seat. Lift out of your hips and lean back over your chair. Let your head move back as you stretch your chin away. You can even sit with your back to the wall and find an angle to rest your head against the wall that provides complete relaxation.

Take the arms overhead and stretch them away like two rays of energy, to expand the backbend and make this stretch more invigorating. Take care that you do not slump—keep each vertebra actively lifting away from the one below it. Take five to ten chest-opening breaths.

## CENTERING

Sit comfortably on your chair. Have your feet well anchored to the ground. Bring the backs of your hands to your thighs. Sit with your back erect so you are not leaning against the back rest. Let your arms and shoulders relax and have your chin parallel to the floor. With each inhalation observe the expansion of the abdomen, ribs and chest. The whole torso is alive with the gentle pulsation of the breath. Even the back of the body opens up, then softens inward rhythmically. Raise the inhalation from the back of the waist, upward. Each time you exhale feel the natural, passive release. As all heavy thoughts float away, the head will lighten so it feels like it's floating happily on the top of your spine. The more you practice this, the quicker you will learn to re-center. Do it whenever you can throughout the day, letting tensions drift away as you return to your true, peaceful inner self.

# RELAXING FORWARD BEND

Sit on the chair with your feet body-width apart. If your feet don't touch the floor easily, place a telephone directory underfoot. Fold forward with a flat back to lay your ribs on your thighs. Like a rag doll, your arms hang out of their sockets, backs of the hands on the floor, fingers softly curled. Your upper body grows heavier. Completely let go of your head and shoulders so they release down toward the floor. Any worries drop away. Now deepen the breath, so the front of your torso expands into the thighs and the space between them. Follow your exhalation for its entire length and observe how it lengthens effortlessly. Stay like this one to five minutes before slowly coming up.

# TWIST

Sit with your left hip to the back of the chair. Have your knees and feet hip-width apart. Rest your feet on a support if they don't easily meet the ground. Raise your arms straight up in the air. Let your torso rise out of your hips. Keep this lift as you twist around to the left and hold the back of the chair. Work from a steady base by keeping your hips and knees level. Twist progressively up the spine. Stay for ten breaths before changing sides.

# PALMING

Refresh with your own portable eyebag. Rub your hands together so the friction builds heat. Rest your elbows onto your desk and rest your head into your hands, palms over your closed eyes. Lean forward to apply a gentle pressure to your eyelids. Withdraw into yourself and observe the wavelike rhythm of your breath.

# SHOULDER STRETCHES

The arm positions of Gomukhasana (see page 64), and Garudasana (see page 98) can easily be practiced in a chair and are great for those working in offices.

# EXPLORE

Your body wants to move. It was made for it! Stretch anytime using the poles at bus stops, walls or by grasping doorways to hang forward to open the chest. While watching TV, sit on floor and notice that you will naturally want to stretch when you change positions. Sit in front of the sofa and use it as a back support for squatting or Cobbler's Pose (see page 60).

# PRANAYAMA

# PRANAYAMA

Have you ever watched children in the playground and marvelled at their never-ending energy? Have you ever felt that you were more tired than you should have been—as if the equation of energy expenditure versus remaining energy didn't add up?

People usually nominate food as the provider of our energy but we forget about a couple of other important sources. Ideas, for one, supply us with boundless energy. You may have experienced being so taken with an idea that you were able to work late into the night without feeling fatigued. A third energy source, recognized by yogis for millennia, is the breath.

Breath, life and energy are rooted together and yogis have a single word for all three—"prana." Yogis consider death to occur when prana, the vital force, leaves the body. Conversely, when pranic levels are high, the body will be completely charged with energy. Pranayama may be translated either as restraint or control of the breath, or as pranic capacity. Pranayama exercises use breathing techniques to increase vitality and mental focus, and to expand consciousness.

Now become aware of your breath. Maintain this awareness until you have finished reading this introduction.

We don't have to think to breathe; it is instinctive and happens automatically. The breath is usually under the control of the medulla oblongata in the relatively primitive brain stem. During pranayama breathing, it shifts from being an involuntary and automatic process toward being more of a voluntary one, and it seems this activates the cerebral cortex, a more evolved part of the brain. Pranayama, by bringing a voluntary element to this involuntary process, has profound physiological, psychological, and spiritual effects.

Most simply, a breath is an intake of oxygen that gets distributed to our cells. The efficient, natural breath ensures that every cell in your body receives the energy it needs to do its job: digest, grow, heal, detoxify. Logically, a healthy body will be composed of well-nourished cells. Deep, conscious breathing, which fully expands the lungs, has an enormously positive impact on health and enhances all cellular processes. When we breathe better, we feel better.

When you touch a baby's belly, or a kitten's or puppy's, you can feel the whole torso moving completely freely. The chest and belly open and blossom with each breath. There is a delightful inner pulsation from expansion to consolidation, a sense of real freedom. However, as we move through life, we inevitably sustain some blows. Particularly as children, we have a limited capacity to understand. In response to the impacts of life, we form shielding patterns in our bodies. At some points, in some areas, our breath ceases to be the joyfully free flow it once was, and deviates into a new protective pattern. As adults we still breathe automatically and unconsciously, but due to our reactions to life, few of us breathe optimally. Those energetic children we were watching in the playground most likely still have relatively free breathing, responsive to the natural cues of the body.

Everything we do is affected by our breathing. The breath and the mind are intrinsically related; they are two expressions of the same entity. Think of the last time you felt angry or fearful: your breath became fast, shallow, and irregular. Compare this to when you were dozing in a comfortable chair. Probably your breath was deeper and slower. Just as your mind affects the breath, your breath affects the mind. Yogis have long recognized that when the breath becomes calm, the mind will too. The *Hatha Yoga Pradipika*, an ancient text, tells us, "Respiration being disturbed, the mind becomes disturbed. By restraining respiration (pranayama), the Yogi attains steadiness of the mind."

The breath is a bridge to our nervous system, and enhanced breathing can improve our mental and emotional states. Firstly, by simply observing our breathing, we gain a mental point of focus that can quiet the constant chatter of the mind. Secondly, it relaxes the mind to promote clear thinking, decrease emotional fluctuations and provide a sense of wellbeing. It is a valuable tool for self-management. Thirdly, like meditation, pranayama draws the senses inward, deepens awareness, and expands consciousness.

Conscious breathing encourages conscious action and conscious living in a calmer way. For returning to the self, we have been given the miracle of the breath. A good breathing habit is a wonderful ally in life, a valuable tool for self-management when dealing with confrontations, fear, agitation, anger, and confusion. Conscious breathing is certainly a mental challenge. Did you remember to be aware of your breath even as you were sitting reading?

## ABOUT PRACTICING

The exercises fall into two categories. During exercises in returning to the natural breath (*see* pages 28 and 132), you immerse yourself in your true breath and begin to disentangle it from any other superimposed breathing patterns. These exercises, where you don't add anything to your breath, are a great starting place. Release any pressure you may feel to breathe "correctly" or do it "the right way" and let your instincts take over. You can repeat them every day for weeks or months to get to know your breath, and return to them as often as you wish. The remaining exercises are pranayama, some of which lead on to more advanced practices involving alteration of the breath. If you wish to develop these practices further, the best way is to work alongside an experienced teacher.

Breath awareness and pranayama are fundamental. Ideally, they should be practiced daily. Just a few minutes will still be worthwhile. Use Savasana relaxation (*see* page 22) to separate pranayama and asana practice so that your energies settle.

## CAUTION

Very deep inhalations should not be practiced if you have hypertension or heart problems. Extremely long exhalations are not advisable if you suffer from low blood pressure or depression.

# HOW TO SIT

Our bodies are as individual as our personalities, so no single position reigns supreme for pranayama or meditation. There are really only two rules for sitting. The first is to sit erect so that your head, neck and back are in line. The second is to be perfectly comfortable. Any physical discomfort will interfere with your concentration, alter your breath, and undo a little of your good work.

One of the things that make pranayama special is that everyone can do it. If you can breathe, you can practice yoga! If you are ill or weak, lie down. You could use the breathing bed (see page 24) or, alternatively, let the torso soften down by lying flat and placing a bolster under your knees. Better still, keep yourself from drifting off to sleep by bending your knees, placing your feet on the floor a little wider than your hips, and letting the knees lean in together. If you find yourself getting sleepy, separate the knees.

## SUKHASANA
**Comfortable Pose**

Before practicing the cross-legged postures, use the leg cradling warm-up (see page 56) to unwind the leg at the hip socket. For Sukhasana, sit cross-legged and slide your feet apart so that each foot comes to rest underneath the opposite knee. It is difficult to sit upright with your shoulders over your hips if your knees are much higher than your hips. Use cushions or folded blankets to raise your seat if necessary.

## VAJARASANA Firm Pose

Kneel with your knees and ankles together and sit down on your heels. As you bring your weight down, your inner ankles will tend to splay apart. Keep them as close together as possible. If it causes discomfort for the tops of the feet, place a small rolled blanket under them. If you like, you can place a folded blanket over your heels before sitting down.

## SITTING IN A CHAIR

Sit a little away from the back rest so your spine will be straight. If your feet don't easily touch the ground, rest them on a rolled blanket or telephone book. Fold a blanket several times to make a long pad. Experiment with it lying across the knees in any of these poses. By placing the backs of your hands on the support, your elbows will bend more and softness will come into the palms.

## SIDDHASANA Perfect Pose

Sit on a cushioned surface. Fold one leg in so the heel touches to the perineum—the area between the anus and the genitals. Bend the second leg and bring the heel of that foot level with the first one. Rest the backs of your hands on your knees.

# UJJAYI PRANAYAMA

## VICTORIOUS BREATH

*Uj* comes from the word for "up" and *jaya* means "triumph" or "conquest." Become victorious over any imbalance in the upward-moving prana with Ujjayi breathing. As you grow more comfortable with Ujjayi breathing, use it for the duration of your asana practice.

Ujjayi breathing is a little like drinking air through a straw. The glottis lies just behind the larynx, near the male Adam's apple. It's the part of the throat that closes when you gargle or hold your breath. As the air flows past the partially closed glottis, friction is produced. This friction increases heat in the body, allowing it to stretch more than it otherwise would during yoga asana practice. Ujjayi breathing thins the breath, giving control over the flow of air into the lungs so that the breath becomes steadier, deeper and longer. More oxygen is made available, enhancing the purification and nourishment of each and every cell.

**1.** Sit in your meditative position. Breathe in through the nose and out through the mouth. Each time you exhale, make a long "haaaa" sound through your mouth, as if you were trying to fog up a mirror.

**2.** After several cycles, close your mouth midway through an exhalation, but continue to make the "haaaa" with your lips together. It will become a soft sound like a "hm" that you can feel in the back of the throat. To check if you've got it, cover your ears with your palms and listen to the internal throaty sound. It will sound like the ocean.

**3.** Now bring it into the inhalation. Open your mouth again and make this "haaaa" sound as you suck in the air. Close your mouth midway through to experience the soft, throaty friction again.

When you feel you have got it, cover your ears to check the ocean-like quality of the sound.

**4.** Now you are ready for the continuous internal "hm" breathing with your mouth closed. At first, practice Ujjayi for 10 to 20 breaths while sitting. Take breaks to return to your natural breath whenever you need. This breath is soft in nature and volume. The sound provides a point of focus for your internalized awareness. It's not necessary to breathe loudly or aggressively. While the sound produced is audible to someone close by, it's not necessary to fill the whole room. Measure the quality of your Ujjayi breathing, not by volume, but by length and steadiness. Bring your awareness to the constancy that this breath gives you. There should be no surges in the breath. It should be clean, even, and pleasant. Each inhalation extends in a long, fluid way to fill the lungs completely. Likewise, the flow of air through your nostrils is slow and steady for the entire duration of the exhalation.

## EXPLORE

A few rounds of Ujjayi will center you whenever you like. You can practice it whenever you are tense, or while out walking. Using Ujjayi breathing during your yoga asana practice will focus your mind.

# DISCOVERING THE BREATH

## BREATHING IN ALL DIRECTIONS

This exercise is usually done with a partner, but can also be done alone. Lightly place your own hands where a partner's hands would be. Then let your shoulders slide up and elbows fall down toward the floor as you curl your palms around your sides. Alternatively, you can hug yourself, placing your hands below your armpits. Finally, let your elbows and shoulders be as heavy and relaxed as possible, as you place your hands on your back ribs. Helpers can direct their breath to the same areas as their partner. You may find that you both begin to breathe in time.

## BREATHING INTO THE FRONT

**1.** Lie on your back with your knees bent and feet flat on the floor. With feet wider than hips, lean your knees together. Helpers need to be sitting perfectly comfortably so they can hold the position for the duration. Any tension will spill over to their partner. Your helper places one palm over your navel and the other high up on the chest, little finger just below the notch at the base of the throat, using a light touch to increase awareness. Have your partner read the instructions, with generous pauses after each sentence to allow you to explore.

**2.** Close your eyes. Observe how your body moves with each inhalation. Which part of your body moves first? Can you feel where the breath originates? What happens next? Observe the sequence of movement. What happens to the lower and upper abdomen? How does the ribcage alter? And the chest? Which part feels like it expands more? Let the breath move you. What happens to the shoulders, the throat? Is there any tightness or constriction there? What about the face and nostrils?

**3.** Now turn your attention to the out breath. From where does your exhalation begin? Where does your exhalation end? Are the movements in the torso as clearly demarcated as in your inhalation? There is a yielding quality to the exhalation, a slow release as the body softens down into the floor. Can you feel a sort of consolidation in toward the center of your torso as you exhale? Could it be that the exhalation ends prematurely? Can you extend the exhalation by being patient and not rushing on to the next breath?

## BREATHING INTO THE SIDES

**1.** Maintain the quiet stillness as your partner changes position to hold the side ribs, cupping just under the armpits. Observe the horizontal expansion of the ribs on the inhalation; the outward and upward movement each time you draw air in. If you don't feel much movement, exhale more fully so that the inhalation naturally deepens. Observe how each exhalation brings a downward and inward movement.

**2.** Now pay attention to the timing of these movements in relation to your abdomen and chest. As you inhale, you might find the abdomen expands first, then the side ribs move up and out and, finally, the upper chest expands. If this movement is difficult to isolate, then you should momentarily try to deepen your breathing so that you can discover your particular pattern. What is your pattern of breathing out? Can you isolate the order of movement of the abdomen, side ribs, and chest, or do they seem to run together?

# BREATHING INTO THE BACK

**1.** Keeping your mental focus, kneel and fold forward into Child Pose. You need to be completely comfortable, so for modifications of the posture *see* page 21. Your partner places their hands just below your shoulder blades, fingers wrapping around the sides.

**2.** Take your breath to the back of your body. Mentally direct the air into your partner's hands. As if you had little balloons under your partner's hands, feel your inhalation "puff" out against them. Have patience as you wait for the movement to come. Many people find this rather difficult and developing this awareness may take several practices.

**3.** In the beginning, you might find it helpful to limit your breathing into the front of the torso by slightly holding in the part of the abdomen below the navel. Visualize the breath moving into the back of the body. As well, have your partner press in slightly during your exhalation to remind you where to expand out to on the inhalation. Once you begin to get a feeling for it, you will feel the whole back come alive. It opens and blossoms with each inhalation, before softening down on each exhalation.

# EXPLORE

Once you are able to isolate breathing into the back, you can take the breath up the spine. Each time you inhale, visualize the inhalation starting at the base of the spine and moving all the way up toward the head. Each inhalation energizes the spine, and each exhalation consolidates that energy, filling the body with prana.

# BHRAMARI HUMMING BEE BREATH

## 48

Making sounds is a great way to bring constancy to the breath. It also lengthens the exhalation, which will naturally deepen the inhalation and encourage a slow, rhythmic breath. Don't be shy of making a sound out loud. The sound provides a point of focus for the mind. As the *Hatha Yoga Pradipika* states, "By this practice one becomes lord of the yogis and the mind is absorbed in bliss." Lose yourself in the vibrations and simply enjoy the soothing effect of Bhramari on the mind.

**1.** Sit comfortably erect, or lie with your knees bent up. Have your mouth closed, jaw relaxed and the teeth slightly apart. Pressing your tongue lightly to the roof of the mouth will create a slight tension and turn the simple humming more into a bee-like droning.

**2.** Inhale fully, then exhale while making a humming sound. The vocal cords keep just a small amount of tension so the pitch is low. The constancy of the exhalation keeps the sound uniform. The vibration comes from the soft palate at the top of the back of the mouth. Widen the inside of the mouth to increase the resonance in the nasal cavity. Hone your awareness of the vibration to expand it out to the throat, to the top of the head, and eventually to the rest of the body. Practice Bhramari for two minutes and build to five. Afterward, sit or lie quietly with eyes closed to enjoy the after-effects. Should you experience dizziness or tingling, or should your mind become agitated, switch to simple breathing.

**3.** Another position for practice is sitting on a blanket with your knees bent up in front of you. Place your elbows on your knees so you can easily cover your eyes with your hands and the flap over your ear holes with your thumbs. Become absorbed in the sound that seems to fill the skull.

3

## EXPLORE

Don't let stress creep in during any breathing exercise. Trying "too hard" changes the lungs, diaphragm, and nervous system, which in turn will adversely affect your body and mind. Evenness in the breath will lead to evenness of temperament.

# MEDITATION

# MEDITATION

Gazing at the sun with wide-open eyes blinds the vision. If you don't stare at it directly, but instead look away a little, you can get a sense of it. Meditation is like that. A change of focus reduces the glare of superfluous distractions and helps us see past the false perceptions to contact the peace and happiness that reside within.

Meditation quietens the mind. Of the eight limbs of Yoga, it is placed seventh, close to the culmination of the state of Yoga—the cessation of all the fluctuations of the thoughts. During meditation, we open up the space between the end of one thought and the beginning of the new one.

Meditators do not tune out life's challenges. Rather, they gain greater insight into their perceptions and their response to stressful situations. As the brain patterns merge into the "theta state"—deeper than sleep—the meditator experiences a state of restful alertness: fully conscious and aware. In meditation we practice being the observer, not the doer. We observe our thoughts and remain detached, without altering the thought patterns at all. Remaining neutral toward our thoughts means that we do not lend them energy to disturb the mind. Whereas before you might have been seeing yourself and the world in a dusty mirror, meditation helps to wipe the mirror clean for new perceptions and true reflections.

## STUDIES—BLOOD PRESSURE

Many studies have been done on meditation, particularly Transcendental Meditation (TM), which involves meditation using a mantra for 20 minutes, twice a day. A study made in 1996 on hypertensive African-Americans in California found that TM significantly lowered blood pressure—more than did any other relaxation technique or education and lifestyle changes. Those who practiced TM for three months saw an average reduction of 10 to 12 points in systolic blood pressure and six to eight points in diastolic pressure (similar results to those of antihypertensive drugs). Through meditation, participants had decreased their risk of heart attack by 11 percent, and stroke by 8–15 percent.

## STRESS AND RELATED DISEASES

Researchers at Harvard Medical School used MRI technology to monitor brain activity on meditators. They found that meditation activates the sections of the brain in charge of the autonomic nervous system. This governs the functions in our bodies that we can't control, such as digestion and blood pressure. As these functions are often compromised by stress, it could mean that by lessening the adrenaline surges as a response to stress, meditation would decrease stress-related conditions, such as hypertension, heart disease, asthma, insomnia, digestive problems, and so on.

A study on stress levels was published in the *American Journal of Health Promotion*. Sixty-two people who reported abnormally high levels of stress participated. Twenty-seven people were the control group. Thirty-five underwent 28 hours of "mindfulness training" involving meditation, yoga postures, and stress-relief techniques over two months. After three months, the mindfulness trainees reported a 54 percent drop in psychological distress, as well as a 46 percent reduction in medical symptoms. The control group reported no improvement in psychological symptoms and a slight increase in medical complaints.

## HEALING

The word "meditation" comes from the Latin root *meditor*, which literally means "healing," and meditation has been found to reduce costs in health care. In Canada, researchers tracked a group of 677 people enrolled in a health insurance program. After learning TM, their health care payments were reduced by 5–7 percent cumulatively every year. After seven years, health costs had been cut by almost 50 percent. Another study of health insurance statistics was published in *Psychosomatic Medicine*. It studied more than 2,000 people practicing TM over a five-year period. It found they had 50 percent fewer doctors' visits and fewer than half the hospitalizations than other groups of similar age, profession, and insurance coverage. Meditators had fewer incidents of illness in 17 categories, including 87 percent fewer hospitalizations for heart disease and 55 percent fewer for cancer.

## INTELLIGENCE

A study published in the *British Journal of Personal and Individual Differences* showed that students practicing transcendental meditation increased their IQ by five points in two years and by nine points in four years.

## AGEING

Meditation has even been found to slow ageing. A study in *The International Journal of Neuroscience* found that a group of 50-year-olds who were practicing transcendental meditation for over five years showed a 12-year decrease in "biological age" as compared to controls. And in the words of one old-timer, "Meditators grow older but they don't necessarily have to grow old."

An ancient healer stated "Man is ill, because he is never still." In India, teachers often refer to our monkey-like minds, which flit around randomly. The Vedas, the earliest known compilations of Indian spiritual writings, say the mind is harder to control than the wind. Achieving the cessation of thought patterns is certainly a tall order, but don't be disheartened. Even if you never arrive at this point, enormous benefits can be derived along the path. The Latin root word *meditor* comes from the Sanskrit *madha*, meaning "wisdom." Meditators feel that meditation improves their quality of life and gives them a sense of the inner peace that is at the core of all of us. This superconscious state allows us to re-center. We tap into a positive universal energy, something greater than ourselves. It gives a wonderful feeling of being completely known—like the feeling you have when your beloved has seen all of you, good and bad, and still loves you. Meditation is a source of great inner strength and is something wonderful to come home to.

# YOGAMUDRASANA SEALING POSE

49

This pose quietens the mind and is a good preparation pose for meditation. Alternatively, you can practice becoming absorbed in the breath (*see* page 132) or Bhramari (*see* page 135).

Sit in Siddhasana (see page 130) by first folding your right leg in, then bringing the left heel in front of the right. Grasp your left wrist with your right hand behind your back. Inhale and extend the torso upward, then exhale and fold forward, bringing your forehead to the floor. Rest for at least a minute, observing the breath and the mind. Then, with eyes closed, come up and change sides with the legs and hands before repeating.

For the mind to quieten you need to be physically comfortable. If this seated position does not feel steady and easy, then practice while sitting on the heels. Rest the forehead on a folded blanket if necessary.

## ABOUT MUDRAS

Whereas bandhas (*see* page 10) are powerful energy locks, mudras, or energy seals, act more gently. Yogis believe that mudras stimulate the flow of prana through the body and seal it in so it's not lost. Some mudras are similar to asanas. Others are hand gestures that may be used during pranayama or meditation. A number of mudras are linked with the chakras. If a mudra also involves contraction of the muscles, then it becomes a bandha.

## USEFUL MUDRAS FOR MEDITATION

Mudras influence the subtle bodies and increase receptiveness to higher states of consciousness.

For Gyana Mudra (also called Jnana Mudra) join the tip of the thumb and index fingers while keeping the other fingers straight.

For Bhajrava Mudra (Gesture of Shiva) place your right hand on your left. Rest your hands in your lap, with your palms facing up and let the tips of your thumbs touch.

# HOW TO MEDITATE

A natural time for meditation is at the end of your yoga asana practice, when the body is warm and loose. Otherwise, do a few limbering stretches that release your body and bring you into the present moment. Then follow these six steps.

*Above: Yogamudrasana.*

### 1. Set the Body
You can practice Yogamudrasana (*see* page 140), Discovering the Breath (*see* page 132) or Bhramari breathing (*see* page 135).

*Above: Bhramari breathing.*

*Right: Discovering the breath.*

## 2. Set the Mind

Decide how long you will sit for. Choose a quiet place and turn off the phone. Cover yourself with a blanket or shawl if necessary. Assume your meditative position. Make sure the back, neck, and head are in line. See the pranayama section (page 126) for suggested sitting positions.

Some people like to offer a personal prayer or chant as a little ritual to carry them into the session. In any case, clarify your intention, reminding yourself of your higher goal and your reason for meditating.

## 3. Relax the Body

While seated, mentally check in with each part of the body. Start from your toes and relax everything bit by bit up to the crown of your head. Once relaxed, commit to not moving your body any more. Any physical movement only serves to distract.

## 4. Focus the Mind

The breath is a wonderful tool to deepen concentration. Begin by observing the flow of air through the nostrils. Observe the minute sensations at the nostrils: the cool air as it flows in through the nostrils, and the warmed air that flows out. There is no need to judge your breath or change the way you are breathing. Patiently be aware simply of what is. You are the detached observer. Practicing detachment is useful for the times in life that you are challenged by pain or difficulty. If you like, count your breaths in rounds of ten.

## 5. Expansion of Consciousness

Steer your thoughts to an attitudinal theme or virtue; a hypergoal such as freedom from attachments, inner peace, or spiritual self-realization.

## 6. Finally

To close, repeat a prayer or use a chant if you find it helpful. When your time for sitting has ended, don't jump up and start racing through your day in an automated way. You have just connected with your inner self with a greater force. Stay mindful and carry this sensation through into your daily life and personal relationships.

# MEDITATION TECHNIQUES

Meditation is a deeply personal thing. More than a technique or a practice, meditation is an experience. There is no one way that is better than another. Try out some ways to see what you feel works best for you. After some experimentation, find a technique with which you feel an affinity and stick to it for at least several months.

## CHAKRA MEDITATION

By moving your awareness to the appropriate physical spot on the body, you can meditate on a chakra. Each chakra has a seed sound associated with it, which you can use as a mantra. Alternatively, you may choose to meditate on the pure color of the chakra (see page 150 for chakra mantras and colors).

*Right: Trataka, or steady gazing, will develop into a meditation over time.*

## TRATAKA Steady Gazing

Trataka is a good practice for "dharana," or concentration, the sixth limb of yoga. You may gaze at a lit candle, picture, symbol, or deity to which you feel drawn. Over time, trataka moves from being a concentration exercise to become a meditation.

## MANTRA MEDITATION

Many people derive great benefit from using a mantra. See page 146 for more information on mantras.

## MOVING MEDITATION

Any action performed with mindfulness can be meditative. A walking meditation is useful if you find sitting for long periods very uncomfortable, or if you tend to fall asleep. You might begin sitting, then, when you are ready, stand up. Keep your eyes unfocused, gazing down to the floor. Walk with your awareness on the feet. Feel the sensations in each sole as it rolls down to contact the floor, bears weight, and then peels off the floor to take the next step. Stay keenly focused on the changes in the weight borne by each foot as you slowly walk in a circle. After this walking meditation, sit and continue the meditation.

# THEMED MEDITATIONS

Choose a subject on which you would like to expand your awareness, such as love or peace. During breath or mantra meditation you attempt to confine the thoughts to a single subject—the breath or the mantra. In a themed meditation you can expand your consciousness by further refining the focus: from many thoughts around a subject, you can reduce to a single thought on it.

The aim is not to prevent all thought but to attain a one-pointed awareness. Observe the flow of thought, like ripples in a lake, without following them. If you follow a thought that isn't the focus of your meditation, you are lending it the energy to distract yourself. Practice mastery over the mind and gently bring your mind back to your chosen subject. The constant churning of the mind eventually gives way to peacefulness.

*Right: The aim of meditation is not to prevent all thought but to attain a one-pointed awareness.*

# MORE ON MEDITATION

Set aside a regular time to meditate. Yogis believe the best times of day to meditate are sunrise, noon, sunset, or midnight, but the most important thing is to find a time in your schedule that you know you will be able to stick to. Don't set yourself up for failure by choosing an impossible time. Likewise, decide realistically how long you can dedicate to each meditation. Then keep to it—don't come out of it early. Some people use a timer set to beep gently when the time has elapsed. Traditionally, east- or north-facing positions are considered conducive to spiritual practice.

Sitting perfectly still can become difficult as every physical sensation is magnified. Breathe through itches as they arise. Remind yourself that all things change; these sensations are only transitory, and can provide the energy for better focus. For a busy mind, being mindful—doing nothing except paying attention—gets boring. Instead of inventing things to relieve this boredom, stay with the meditation, accept that you are feeling bored, and make it the subject of your attention for a while.

Although meditation brings people peace, it can also bring to mind other issues. As a process of self-observation, you may be confronted with thoughts or parts of your character that you would prefer not to recognize. Facing certain feelings you are not owning up to can raise your level of anxiety, as if there is nowhere to hide. Although it can be very disturbing, remind yourself that all things change. Becoming aware of your shadow side actually allows you to operate in a different way.

Like your yoga practice, meditation experiences will vary from day to day. Don't classify meditations as "good" or "bad." Perhaps a meditation feels "bad" because it has thrown up something you find uncomfortable. It might feel more difficult but could actually offer you a lot. Try not to become too attached to the highs you experience on your spiritual path. If we cling to these feelings we may miss the point of the exercise, which is a feeling of unity with the universe as a whole. Refrain from judging the highs and lows and simply welcome that experience as part of the unceasing flow of life.

In meditation, we often seek to encourage a detachment from worldly things. While this type of detachment can assist us in objective observation, it does not mean that we should stop caring about what happens to the world. We need to continue interacting in an open-minded and loving way.

# MANTRAS AND CHANTING

A mantra is a potent sound that helps harmonize the system, a vibrational force that carries healing. Reciting a mantra or devotional verse in a yogic chant is uplifting and soothing.

## MANTRA

A mantra can be a syllable, a word or a phrase that is generally repeated over and over. Using a mantra provides a point of focus for the mind. A mantra is a positive affirmation: a constant reminder and a way to bring yourself back to base. Reciting a mantra is an exercise in dharana (concentration) that can become dhyana (meditation).

Many mantras are in the ancient language of Sanskrit. Sanskrit is made up of primordial sounds and each syllable creates a particular resonance within the body. A Sanskrit mantra is a particular combination of sound vibrations that, when chanted or meditated upon, has a specific effect on the body, mind, and psyche. This resonance assists healing and spiritual elevation. In each repetition a certain energetic vibration is being sent out into the world. For this reason the pronunciation needs to be spot on, so if you are not sure, ask a yoga teacher about the correct pronunciation for your mantra.

Though traditionally given by a guru, you can certainly choose your own mantra. It is not necessary to have an exotic-sounding mantra. You may feel more affinity with a mantra in your own language such as peace, love, or faith.

If you would like to use a mantra for meditation, you can begin each session by chanting the mantra aloud and letting the resonance flow through the body. Then, keeping the reverberation, take the volume down to a whisper and, finally, continue your meditation by repeating it mentally.

Mantra is often used at the beginning and end of a yoga class. It can be as simple as chanting *om* three times with the teacher. You can link your mantra practice to work with particular areas of the body and the chakras (*see* page 150). Many people find using a mantra helps in times of stress—even in public places a mantra can be repeated silently. Like an affirmation, it's a helpful reminder to bring you back to base.

## SOME COMMON MANTRAS

*Om*—This sacred syllable is considered the mother of all sounds. As with other Sanskrit mantras, it is believed that it sets up a special vibration in your body and mind, and this is spread out into the world. It is used by both Hindus and Buddhists. *Om* is composed of the three sounds A-U-Mmmm running together. The first "A" sound will resonate more in the belly. The "U" moves the vibration up to the chest cavity. The final long "M" sound is made into a nasal sound so its resonance is felt more in the head.

**Om namah shivaya**—This is a salutation to the Hindu deity Shiva. Non-Hindus use this mantra, too, intending it to honor the divine in oneself.
**Soham**—This mantra also honors the divine within. Pronounced so-hum, it means "I am the universal self."
**Shanti**—Means "peace" in Sanskrit.
**Om namo bhagavate vasudevaya**—Means salutations to the Divine Source, the indweller of all.

# CHANTING

Though some adults feel shy about making sounds out loud, chanting is really perfectly natural. Let go of worrying about how good or bad you sound. Chanting is not like singing but more like reciting. The purpose is not to have the most beautiful voice, but rather to feel the sound resonate through the body.

The devotional path of yoga is called Bhakti Yoga where God or God's representative spiritual teacher is worshipped. In Bhakti Yoga, spiritual verses are chanted with fervent devotion. There is a sense of connection to something greater than the self, as the heart center opens up to a crescendo of universal love. Then the emotions are settled down to stabilize once more. This climax and settling of the emotions is similar to a heartbroken person crying out a song about lost love. When the emotions are relived in a small way, then left to settle, it's very healing on the emotional sphere.

Even if you don't consider yourself religious, chanting can be a worthwhile and fulfilling experience. A chanting session is incredibly soothing. It feels like a balm for the brain. It seems to wipe away all the usual preoccupations, so it's like taking an instant mental holiday. In addition, it clarifies your intentions and is uplifting for the heart. If you are not comfortable with a chant to God, you may feel more comfortable interpreting it as being a chant to the light you carry within. If you ask around, you may find a chanting group in your area.

## CHANTS TO START AND FINISH YOUR YOGA PRACTICE

*Om asathoma sadgamaya*
*Thamasoma Jyotirgamaya*
*Mrithyorma Amrithangamaya*
*Om Shanti Shanti Shanti*

*Om Lead me from the unreal to the real*
*From darkness to light*
*From the predicament of death to immortality*
*Om peace, peace, peace*

*Om*
*Swasthi praja bhyah pari pala yantam*
*Nya yena margena mahi mahi shaha*
*Go brahmanebhyaha shubhamastu nityam*
*Lokaa samastha sukhino bhavantu*
*Om*

*Om*
*Let prosperity be glorified*
*Let rulers rule the world with law and justice*
*Let divinity and wisdom be protected*
*Let people of the world be happy and prosperous*
*Om*

# THE KUNDALINI PATH

# CHAKRAS

Hatha Yoga exercises focus on the vertebral column and work not only on the physical body but also on the subtle bodies. The twisting, lengthening, and bending forward, backward, and sideways of Hatha Yoga aim to awaken and balance the subtle energies.

According to the yogic tradition, there are many thousands of "nadis"—energy meridians—in our bodies. The largest one is called the Sushumna Nadi. It is not recognized by Western anatomy but it follows a nervous pathway, running from the perineum up the length of the vertebral column.

Yogis speak of a reservoir of energy known as the "kundalini," which resides in the body. Literally translated as "she who is coiled," the kundalini force is likened to a serpent lying dormant at the base of the spine. Yoga exercises seek to undo any energy blockages of the spine, and purify the body and mind to clear the way for this cosmic power to rise. Another way to clear the kundalini path is to work with the chakras.

The word *chakra* means "wheel" in Sanskrit. A chakra, like a wheel or vortex, is an area of increased energy (prana). As a center of energy, a chakra can exist anywhere in the body, though we tend to recognize seven main ones located at various levels up the spine. It is said that the chakras act as transformers. As each chakra has a related nerve and endocrine plexus, they are believed to channel the pranic energy into the physical body at the points of the chakras. It is thought that when all the chakras are fully functioning, the kundalini power can move unimpeded up the body's central energy channel from the base of the spine to the crown of the head. As the kundalini "serpent" uncoils and rises, it enlivens each chakra in turn. When it reaches the top chakra, it is said that a change of consciousness occurs, special psychic powers are obtained and liberation of the soul (the ultimate goal of yoga) is attained.

Each of these seven reservoirs of energy has its own physical, emotional, and spiritual effects. The lower chakras from the base of the spine to the solar plexus are considered to be more physical than the chakras located from the heart to the crown of the head. Many people choose to focus their work on the higher chakras, believing them to be more "spiritual" than the more earthy lower ones. However, like building a house, each level needs to be supported by a solid base below it. The grounding forces of the lower chakras provide the vital steady foundation for balanced spiritual exploration. Should a chakra be out of balance, yoga can help stimulate the less active chakras and move energy along from areas where it is congested, therefore balancing the system. Knowledge of the chakras allows us to understand ourselves a little more; yoga postures are tools with which to facilitate transformation.

# 1 MULADHARA CHAKRA— ROOT CHAKRA

## Location

The base of the spine is the home of the first chakra. The related organs are the organs of elimination and excretion—the lungs, skin, kidneys, large intestine, and rectum.

## Expression

The root chakra governs your connection to the earth and how "rooted" you feel. It deals with your material and monetary existence. It is the chakra that is concerned with getting your basic needs met—like obtaining food, shelter, and even love. It is very involved with how stable you feel emotionally and in your physical set-up. The root chakra is expressed in your strength and stamina. It gives you the drive to get up and go to work in the morning. It allows you to focus, be disciplined, stay healthy, and be aware of your limits.

The root chakra must be balanced as a foundation to balancing the other chakras or your progression will be without roots and stability. When the muladhara chakra is out of balance, it may cause problems of the lower abdominal area, such as constipation, diarrhoea, haemorrhoids, kidney problems, sciatica, and back pain.

As the base chakra has such a grounding force, the psychological impact of imbalance at the level of this chakra can swing from being too grounded to not being grounded enough. A lack of grounding could cause you to live in a fantasy world and feel off-center. You could experience difficulty focusing, or find you go out of control easily. You may find it hard to contain your feelings. On the other hand there may be too much holding on, for example, if you are excessively materialistic or unable to let go of things emotionally. It might manifest itself in being overly controlling and trying to keep a hold over others.

The muladhara chakra is the driving force behind the energy to work. When this chakra is not in balance, you could become overly attached to your work, leading to a workaholic lifestyle. Another manifestation could be diminished creative power, which will interfere with your ability to enjoy life and prevent you from opening up to feelings of joy and happiness.

Aggressiveness and stubbornness can be further signs, as can a tendency toward selfishness, creating material and emotional possessiveness. An imbalance in the root chakra can make you self-serving and self-centered. When your survival is threatened, you feel afraid. This fear can be immobilizing and ultimately prevent you from achieving your goals. The root chakra is awakened when you confront your fears.

When the root chakra is functioning well, there will be good general health for the related organs, like the kidneys and bowel. The adrenal glands, involved in the response to stress, will be healthy, not exhausted from chronic overstimulation. There will be a cheerful, fearless, and courageous attitude. A balanced base chakra brings self-confidence, enthusiasm, a strong will to live, and a clear sense of identity. Trust in others comes easily.

You will have a good perspective on life and be able to stay in touch with the greater scheme of things. You will be able to detach from an overemphasis on the importance of material possessions. There will be a healthy attitude to work. While you will remain focused, you will not be so attached to your work that you ignore other parts of your life. You will approach your work and challenges with enthusiasm and joy. With this attitude, material success can come to you more easily.

# 2 SVADHISTHANA CHAKRA—SEXUAL CHAKRA

## Location

The second chakra is located at the lower abdomen between the navel and the genitals. The second chakra governs the organs of the lower abdominal area, such as those of the urinary and reproductive systems.

## Expression

Its location is a clue that the second chakra is involved with sexuality, relationships, and creativity. The svadhisthana chakra governs our nurturing abilities, and our sensation and pleasure focus. It is also highly involved in relationships, and this includes your relationship with yourself.

Change is an inescapable fact of life. Without change, there is no growth, no movement, no life. The sexual chakra is connected with change and how you deal with it. A well-balanced second chakra allows you to go with the flow and alter your path as necessary.

If you have an imbalance in this chakra, it could affect the urinary, reproductive, and circulatory systems. Impotence, sexually transmitted diseases, and bladder problems could be signs that the second chakra needs some attention.

People who have an unbalanced sexual chakra have difficulty with giving or receiving materially or emotionally. Obesity can be a result of a lack of balance between giving and receiving. An overweight person who is consuming more calories than they are using is taking more than they are giving. The second chakra helps with assimilation of knowledge. On the mental level, receiving is linked with the integration of knowledge as the brain takes in and stores information.

Feelings of guilt, anxiety, unpredictability, and clinging on can be an indication of an unbalanced second chakra. Some people may have difficulty separating their own feelings from those of others. General low energy or lack of creativity can also be connected to this chakra. Sexual desire may be too little or too much. Flirting outrageously or using sex to gain attention are further signs that the chakra is off-balance. A person may become trapped in an unhealthy pattern of seeking excessive sensual pleasure.

A well-balanced second chakra gives a high level of general vitality. The lower abdominal, urinary, and reproductive systems will be healthy. If this chakra is balanced, you will be outgoing, patient and have a good sense of humour. You will be comfortable with your sexuality and content with yourself. You find it easy to be positive and enjoy life.

A main force of this chakra governs the attraction of opposites. There is an unceasing dance between dualities. Movement is created and you can easily go with the flow of life. At the same time, you have intellectual ideas about the world and how your desires and emotions fit in it.

Creative problem-solving and the ability to work creatively with others will come easily. Even if other people have different ideas from you, you are able to work out a complementary path. Rather than forming obstacles, the different approaches and attitudes of others enrich your life and allow you to develop and grow.

# 3 MANIPURA CHAKRA— SOLAR PLEXUS

## Location

The third chakra is situated between the bottom of the breastbone and the navel. It controls the digestive system and related organs, including the liver, stomach, gall bladder, pancreas, spleen, and the organs of excretion.

## Expression

Through its closeness to the digestive system, this third chakra is involved in the production and storage of energy—the same energy that allows us to live our lives effectively. The manipura chakra relates to emotions, actions, power, and will. It helps us recognize that, with effort and action, we can achieve what we want.

The solar plexus center links to your level of comfort with power, and this includes your sense of personal power. Your power comes through being able to bring things together. Rather than seeing things as separate and unrelated, and subdividing them, you are able to find the power in unification. A balanced third chakra helps you develop a healthy will and autonomy. When unbalanced, you may feel powerless, have lower self-esteem and be more easily swayed by the opinions of those around you.

If your third chakra is not in balance, you can experience uncontrolled extreme emotions, such as violent passions, jealousies, anger, and frustration, and they can then turn into doubts, fears, and confusion. There may be a tendency to try to manipulate others. Obsessive characteristics or a tendency to an addictive personality might appear.

Failure to learn to assert your own autonomy can cause you to feel powerless or victimized. With an unbalanced third chakra, you risk running out of emotional steam. Apathy and lethargy cause your energy to turn in on itself and make you want to withdraw from life. You can become overly critical of yourself, causing you to lose the ability to connect and be nourished by your surroundings. Low self-esteem makes you doubt yourself and you can suffer self-recrimination.

There can also be an imbalance of fiery energy. This may manifest itself as feeling hot, avoiding spicy foods, wanting cold drinks, sweating easily or being quick-tempered. Too little fire, on the other hand, can cause you to feel cold, crave hot, spicy foods and hot drinks, or feel slow and lethargic. Any of the related organs might show symptoms. Internally, ulcers, upset stomach, diabetes, hypoglycaemia, or even alcoholism, and, externally, a tight hard belly, large pot-belly, or a sunken diaphragm, may all indicate an imbalance.

A well-balanced manipura chakra gives a great deal of energy, which might show up as having a warm body and fast metabolism. This energy brings an enthusiasm for work, play, development, and transformation in your life. You will feel bright and extroverted and have clear thinking.

You will have a constructive use of power and it will be directed inward, toward the self, instead of being wielded over others. This internal willpower creates proactive, assertive, and confident qualities. Your self-esteem is at a healthy level and there will be a drive toward a consciously controlled positive change, as opposed to passively waiting or wishing for something great to happen. You will be self-motivated and self-accepting. You will be naturally aware of your social responsibility and will approach things from a social perspective. You aren't tempted to abuse your power to manipulate others. Your power is used to bring people and things together, rather than to drive them apart. A balanced manipura chakra produces an inner strength allowing you to perform actions with ease and grace.

# 4 ANAHATA CHAKRA—HEART CENTER

## Location

Located at the center of the chest, the anahata chakra corresponds to love in the pure, unconditional sense. It encompasses the love of nature and the love of all humanity.

## Expression

Physically, the anahata chakra relates to the heart, the circulatory and respiratory systems, the breasts, chest, and shoulders. The fourth chakra brings together the forces of the first three chakras. The first chakra is about solidity and stability, the second governs change and movement, while the third brings into play acceptance and the forces of the will. When these forces come together, they can then be transformed into energies to achieve higher goals. The heart center is the point of transition between the more grounding lower chakras and the higher, spiritual ones.

The heart chakra deals with social awareness, love and openness, a sense of devotion, peace, forgiveness, acceptance, kindness, and joy. While the second chakra has a unifying force that is oriented more to objects or people, the unifying force of the heart chakra is experienced more as a state of being. It is less involved with sexuality, less materialistic, and more conceptual. It deals with the union and harmonious integration of the self into larger social groups without any loss of true sense of self. The force of the anahata chakra allows us to break out of the limitations of our ego. In transcending the ego we can grow toward something deep and strong. It loosens our boundaries as we experience the joy of love.

Physically, an imbalance in the fourth chakra could result in heart conditions, including high blood pressure, and could cause respiratory conditions, asthma, and arthritis of the arms. Emotionally, you might tend toward feeling a conditional type of love. Perhaps you expect something in return for giving your love, or you could confuse love and sex. You may impose your will over others, and tend to be manipulative. On the other hand, you might be overly selfless, often finding yourself in the role of martyr. An imbalance might lead to a lack of sensitivity, arrogance, selfishness, or feelings of sadness or depression.

When the heart chakra is in balance, the related organs and systems will be healthy. There is a sense of connection with all life, which gives peace, joy, and feelings of unconditional love for all beings. Your relationships will be more balanced and harmonious. Your emotions will be free but not unstable, and they can be clearly and spontaneously expressed. You will be open, willing, and able to live without fear of vulnerability. There will be a good balance between the material things in life and your emotions. Because the heart center has an integrative force, helping us overcome dualities, and because love is the ultimate healing energy, the heart chakra is the center for healing.

# 5 Visuddha Chakra—Throat Center

**Location**

Located level with the base of the throat, the fifth chakra is linked to communication and expression.

**Expression**

As its physical location may suggest, the visuddha chakra corresponds to the neck and organs of the neck, including the voice box and airway in the throat. As the related glands are the thyroid and parathyroid glands, the metabolism of the whole body is affected by the fifth chakra.

The throat chakra is involved in the verbal expression of all the thoughts and feelings encompassed by the lower chakras. It affects our speech and how we express ourselves. It is linked to truth and honesty. This center connects our feelings and intuition with our thoughts, making them enter our consciousness and enabling us to act on them. The throat chakra helps form our future. A need or desire is more easily met once it is expressed, so, in a way, we shape our own futures with verbal communication. Like the second chakra, this fifth chakra is strongly linked to creativity: the formation of speech, communication, and expression is an inherently creative process. The throat chakra moves away from the physicality of the chakras below. Its boundaries are more fluid and less physical, being involved in such things as the sharing of information and ideas.

Problems with the throat chakra can show up physically in sore throats, loss of voice, and neck or throat conditions. An over or underactive thyroid, headaches from neck muscle tension, insomnia, flu, and even cancer could be manifestations of an imbalance in this center. Any difficulty in expression or communication indicates an imbalance of the fifth chakra. You may hold back, either in voicing your opinion or showing your thoughts or feelings. On the other hand, you may dominate conversations and discussions. Perhaps you have difficulty expressing your needs or having them met. You could be critical, tactless, deceitful, judgemental, or harsh-voiced, or may suffer from false pride.

When the throat chakra is in balance, the throat area will be physically healthy. You have effective expression and clear communication of your feelings and ideas, and it can show in your voice, making it clear and pleasant to the ear. Creativity, maturity and inspiration help you deal with yourself and others in an honest, compassionate and tactful way. You can make clear assessments without judging others. Verbal expression is made possible by vibrational rhythms, and the throat chakra is linked to rhythm and the pace at which we lead our lives. You will be able to conduct your life at a regular, easy pace, rather than losing yourself in a hectic and destructive lifestyle. A balanced fifth chakra gives you a sense of serenity and devotion.

# 6 AJNA CHAKRA—THIRD EYE CENTER

**Location**

Located between and just above the eyebrows, the sixth chakra is like a third eye, said to be the seat of wisdom.

**Expression**

The sixth chakra is linked to the brain and nervous system. The ears, nose, eyes, and sinuses relate to it. Lastly, the hormonal system is affected by the sixth chakra through the wide-reaching effects of the pituitary gland in the brain. The information-gathering capability of our sense of sight is very powerful. With a single glance we can take on board an enormous amount of information. Taking our ability to "see" and assess situations further, the sixth chakra becomes involved in the capacity for intuition, imagination, visualization, and even clairvoyance. This intuition is the link between our intellectual and psychic abilities. Being guided from within lies beyond the part of the mind telling us we can't do something and the part telling us we can. Intuition is a line to a force greater than ourselves. Physically, an imbalance in the sixth chakra may manifest in headaches or eye, ear, nose, and sinus conditions. Hormonal imbalances, insomnia, and nervous disorders may appear. Depression may arise. The third eye center is linked to the hormonal glands of the brain, and therefore to levels of the neurotransmitter serotonin, depletion of which has been linked to depression.

On another level, depression might come from having lost touch with your essentially creative self—a lack of ability to use and flow with your creativity. When the sixth chakra is out of balance, you can have problems focusing and concentrating and may feel confused and negative. A lack of direction and intellectual stagnation can be experienced. So many people spend many hours a week in a job that doesn't enhance their life. We need to be enriched by what we do. Make sure your work is in harmony with your beliefs. The sixth chakra can help us determine what will enrich us. Your yoga asana practice is useful as it is a journey on the emotional and intellectual level, which opens you up to listen to your intuitive self and the special language of your body: posture, holding patterns, disease, wellbeing.

When the third eye chakra is in balance, you will be able to observe thoughts and feelings without becoming overly attached to them. You have a good level of direction, devotion and high ideals. You are imaginative and carry within yourself a sense of oneness, a feeling of unity. This sense of integration allows you to overcome anxiety. When the ajna chakra is fully awakened, you experience a mastery of the self, known as self-realization.

# 7 SAHASRARA CHAKRA—CROWN CENTER

## Location
The crown chakra is located at the top of the head, at the "soft spot" that is the anterior fontanel.

## Expression
The brain, the whole nervous system and the pineal gland are in the realm of the crown chakra. The root chakra and the crown chakras have opposite forces. While the root chakra acts as the entry point of human life, the crown acts as an exit point. The crown chakra deals with transcending materialism and letting go of physical attachments. The search for meaning—that all things are part of a larger structure—brings us closer to unity. The seventh chakra gives us a coherent sense of meaning. It relates to the highest state of consciousness. It deals with spiritual enlightenment, self-realization, and God-consciousness. The crown chakra is very important as it is the point where the liberation of the soul arrives. When the sahasrara chakra is fully awakened, there is a fusion of the seven chakras and the experience of boundlessness. At this level of consciousness, there is an awareness of a higher or deeper order that integrates and unifies. It reminds us that, even though the body is finite, the soul is infinite.

Physically, cerebral tumours and increased pressure in the skull can be an indication of an imbalance in the crown center. There could be psychological symptoms like psychoses or neuroses or depression. Insomnia may occur due to the crown chakra's link with the pineal gland, which produces melatonin, vital for healthy sleep. It is also linked to Seasonal Affective Disorder Syndrome (SADS), sufferers of which feel down and depressed during colder seasons of less daylight. Emotionally, you may also experience a sense of isolation from the world. There can be a loss of direction, low energy levels, fatigue, and a tendency toward having a "closed mind." When your crown chakra is in balance, you will feel a sense of unity with others without suffering a loss of your individuality. You will pay well-focused attention to them. There is no distortion, but rather a knowledge born of wisdom or enlightenment. You will follow your own ethical ideals and not be overly influenced by outside forces or the opinions of others.

## CHAKRAS AT A GLANCE

| Chakra | Color | Element | Relates to | Element | Mantra |
|---|---|---|---|---|---|
| Muladhara | Red | Ruby | Stability, Survival, Basic Needs | Earth | Lam |
| Svadhisthana | Orange | Amber | Creativity, Sexuality, Relationships | Water | Vam |
| Manipura | Yellow | Gold | Power, Will, Action | Fire | Ram |
| Anahata | Green | Emerald | Unconditional Love, Self-Healing, Joy | Air | Yam |
| Visuddha | Sky Blue | Sapphire | Communication, Self-Expression, Truth | Ether | Ham |
| Ajna | Indigo | Diamond | Intuition, Wisdom | Pure Essence | Om |
| Sahasrara | Violet | Amethyst | Spiritual Illumination, The Bliss State | Boundlessness | (no mantra) |

| Chakra | Balancing the Chakras—General | Meditation | Affirmation | Asanas |
|---|---|---|---|---|
| Muladhara | Get enough sleep every day and rest when you are tired. Massage is grounding and brings you back to body sensations. Foot massage is good. Eat regularly. Don't skip meals. | You can meditate using the seed mantra for this chakra, Lam. | A useful affirmation for this chakra is to repeat in your mind or out loud about ten times, several times a day, "I stand firmly in my life in a loving and imaginative way." | All the standing postures help balance the root chakra. Tadasana Virabhadrasana I, II, III Garudasana Paschimottanasana Savasana |
| Svadhisthana | Massage can help you to let go of old emotions. Rolfing is a form of massage that can release memories from body tissue. It is deep and can be cathartic. But there are also gentler forms of massage that can release emotions for those who prefer a softer approach. Pranayama can help in letting go of emotions, especially with long exhalations. | You can meditate on the seed sound, Vam. | "I am open to the world and flow easily with changes in my life." | Trikonasana Pavritta Trikonasana Ardha Baddha Padma Paschimottanasana Baddha Konasana Paschimottanasana |
| Manipura | Jogging and power-walking overcome sluggishness. Stomach crunches tone the area. Laughing or physical exercise help release suppressed emotions. Let go of emotional attachments that aren't helping you. Ask yourself what is running smoothly and enjoyably in your life right now. How can you use your will and less effort to achieve your goals? | You can meditate on empowerment or use the seed mantra, Ram. | "I move toward my goals smoothly and enjoyably." | Twists, back arches, and forward stretches will assist the solar plexus chakra. Pavritta Trikonasana Ustrasana Jathara Parivartanasana Paschimottanasana Purvottanasana Balasana |

| Chakra | Balancing the Chakras—General | Meditation | Affirmation | Asanas |
|---|---|---|---|---|
| Anahata | An exercise to open the heart chakra is to sit in a crowded place. Choose a person to focus your mind on. While you sit relaxed and breathing deeply, take your time in observing their body movements, their face, their eyes, and the way they speak. Put aside judgement. With each inhalation, build compassion for this person within you, but let go on each exhalation. | You can meditate on the seed mantra, Yam | "My heart opens with love for all beings." | Virabhadrasana I<br>Anjaneyasana<br>Matsyasana<br>Ustrasana<br>Urdva Dhanurasana<br>Passive opening out twist<br>Balasana |
| Visuddha | Because this chakra operates on the level of vibration, chanting that works with the vibration of sound has a purifying effect. *See* the section on mantras (page 146). The breath can be used to calm the nervous system and enhance the quality of the voice, making it fuller, deeper, and clearer. Practice Bhramari and Ujjayi breathing (*see* pages 131 and 135 respectively). | You can meditate on the seed mantra, Ham, or chant it aloud. | "I communicate honestly and directly." | Matsyasana<br>Ustrasana<br>Setu Bandhasana<br>Sarvangasana<br>Halasana<br>Karnapidasana |
| Ajna | Meditation is key to opening the third eye chakra. Sit in a quiet place and focus on your breathing. Allow your breath to move to the area between and just above the eyebrows. Alternatively, do a color meditation, visualizing in turn each of the colors from the first to seventh chakras. From red, move through orange, yellow, green, blue, indigo, and violet. | The seed sound for this chakra is Om. | "I am open to my inner guidance", or "I follow my inner guidance." | Matsyasana<br>Setu bandhasana<br>Sarvangasana<br>Balasana<br>Sirsasana<br>Yogamudrasana |
| Sahasrara | To activate the crown chakra, live your life with as much awareness as possible. While this is more easily said than done, you can use breath awareness exercises, meditation, affirmation, and asanas to help you. | Meditation taps into the world of the seventh chakra. There is no seed sound for this chakra, though you could chant the ancient sacred sound, Om. | "My soul is boundless and infinite." | Any meditation pose sitting erect with the back, neck, and head in line is beneficial to working with the crown chakra.<br><br>Siddhasana<br>Vajarasana<br>Balasana<br>Sirsasana<br>Sasankasana<br>Yogamudrasana |

# INDEX